Praise for
Hippocrates' Shadow

"A clear-sighted, heartfelt, and humane story of the needless tests and treatments that cripple health care—and how to get rid of them. As a guide to good medicine, it may help us get back to the essence of what good doctors do: be with patients in healing."

—SAMUEL SHEM, M.D.,
author of *The House of God,*
Mount Misery, and *The Spirit of the Place*

"There are few books that I really almost cannot put down, but *Hippocrates' Shadow* is one. A stunning indictment of current medical practice by a hardheaded doc tested in big-city emergency rooms, combat hospitals in Iraq, and at his mom's bedside. If your doctor is this frank with you, you are a very lucky patient, and you are getting a lot better (and sometimes a lot less) treatment than most."

—MELVIN KONNER, M.D., PH.D.,
author of *Becoming a Doctor*

"Dr. Newman's book is insightful and thought-provoking. He teaches the reader about aspects of medicine that many of us, laypeople as well as physicians, do not understand or appreciate, including the imperfection of the 'science' of medicine as well as the progressive loss of the 'art of medicine.' Anyone who wishes to better understand the promise and limitations of medicine should read this book."

—GEOFFREY KURLAND, M.D.,
author of *My Own Medicine:*
A Doctor's Life as a Patient

HIPPOCRATES' SHADOW

DAVID H. NEWMAN

Scribner

NEW YORK LONDON TORONTO SYDNEY

The ideas, procedures, and suggestions in this book are not intended as a substitute for the medical advice of a trained health professional. All matters regarding your health require medical supervision. Consult your physician before adopting the suggestions in this book, as well as about any condition that may require diagnosis or medical attention. The author and publisher disclaim any liability arising directly or indirectly from the use of this book.

SCRIBNER
A Division of Simon & Schuster, Inc.
1230 Avenue of the Americas
New York, NY 10020

First Scribner trade paperback edition September 2009

SCRIBNER and design are registered trademarks of The Gale Group, Inc., used under license by Simon & Schuster, Inc., the publisher of this work.

For information about special discounts for bulk purchases, please contact Simon & Schuster Special Sales: 1-866-506-1949 or business@simonandschuster.com

The Simon & Schuster Speakers Bureau can bring authors to your live event. For more information or to book an event, contact the Simon & Schuster Speakers Bureau at 1-866-248-3049 or visit our website at www.simonspeakers.com.

Designed by Kyoko Watanabe
Text set in Dante MT

Manufactured in the United States of America

1   3   5   7   9   10   8   6   4   2

Library of Congress Control Number: 2008012485

ISBN 978-1-4165-5153-9
ISBN 978-1-4165-5154-6 (pbk)
ISBN 978-1-4165-8029-4 (eBook)

For Mom, Dad, Pie, and Dude

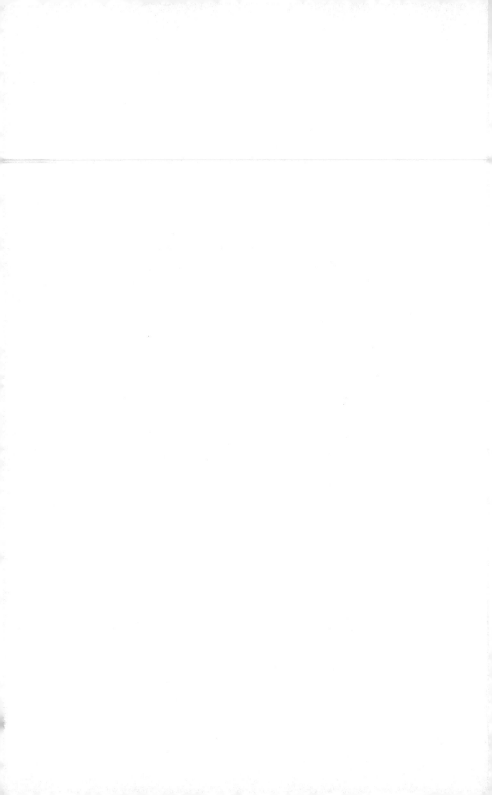

Life is short, the Art long, opportunity fleeting, judgment difficult, experience delusive.

—HIPPOCRATES, 400 B.C.

CONTENTS

HIPPOCRATES'
SHADOW

FOREWORD

Dr. Hippocrates

By today's standards, Hippocrates was a profoundly abnormal physician. Medicine's founding father routinely tasted his patients' urine, sampled their pus and earwax, and smelled and scrutinized their stool. He assessed the stickiness of their sweat and examined their blood, their phlegm, their tears, and their vomit. He became closely acquainted with their general disposition, family, and home, and he studied their facial expressions. In deciding upon a final diagnosis and treatment, Hippocrates recorded and considered dietary habits, the season, the local prevailing winds, the water supply at the patient's residence, and the direction the home faced. He absorbed everything, examining exhaustively and documenting meticulously.

Modern-day physicians often cringe or shake their heads when they hear descriptions of Hippocrates' diagnostic methods; laypeople, however, have quite a different response—they wonder aloud at how nice it might be to have Hippocrates as their doctor. The disparity illustrates the thematic core of this book: somewhere in our twenty-four-hundred-year journey from the island of Cos in ancient Greece to the modern centers of the technologically and scientifically advanced medicine that we now practice, the interests and the goals of patients and doctors have gone their separate ways. Most likely it was at first a subtle divergence, and the chosen road was undoubtedly paved with noble intentions. But no matter how it started, we physicians have steadily moved in a different direction than our patients, and now we are light-years apart.

In 400 B.C., when Hippocrates led the medical academy at Cos, documenting his patient encounters, teaching his students the Art of medicine (he capitalized the *A*), and writing what would become known as the *Hippocratic Corpus,* he was unaware that he was establishing Western medical theory for the next two-plus millennia. But while today's physicians take a lifetime oath adapted directly from his writings, Hippocrates wouldn't recognize our interpretation of the Art.

Hippocrates was a holistic practitioner intent on treating the complete person, whereas today we tend to specialize in exquisitely narrow fields of anatomic and physiologic knowledge, leaving the balance of the human body to our colleagues. Hippocrates was a devoted and objective empiricist, while most modern doctors spend so little time with each patient that it's absurd to claim serious observational skills. Hippocrates was a consummate communicator, while today's doctors (ask our patients) are walking communication nightmares. Hippocrates felt and demonstrated sympathy, while we've chosen a colder, more "scientific" model for doctor-patient interaction. If Hippocrates is the father of the art we now practice, then we are his rebellious, confused, self-centered teenagers.

The fact that patients' and doctors' goals have diverged is apparent to anyone who has been to see a doctor recently. But there is a phenomenon within the culture of modern medicine that guarantees the widening of this patient-doctor chasm. The phenomenon renders true communication virtually impossible, and precludes reconciliation or mutual understanding. Ultimately this phenomenon leads physicians to be aloof and misunderstood—to have, even, a cultlike sense of separation from the rest of humanity. The phenomenon is secrecy. Doctors have secrets, and we have lots of them.

My book is an attempt to reveal those secrets, to halt the masquerade. But this is easier said than done. Not all secrets are easy to expose. Some lie deep in the minds of physicians and are difficult to access (without help), while others are as simple and as clear as the light of day. Some are so obvious that everyone knows them, though few have spoken them aloud. Some are manifest in almost every interaction a doctor has with a patient, while others are specific to a disease, or a condition, or an encounter. There are so many secrets that this book can only begin the process of unveiling.

It is my sincere hope that physicians will read this book and see that it isn't a whistle-blowing exposé designed to vilify individuals or individual groups. The truth is, the real secrets of modern medicine are protected by tradition, group-think, and system constructs that punish inquiry and self-examination. They are embedded in the presumptions and thought patterns that we are taught to embrace during our indoctrination and on which we come to rely. They originate at the highest levels and trickle down; physicians are often merely bit players in a systemic—and systematic—dishonesty stemming from these secrets. These are the secrets and lies that shape the practice of modern medicine.

The situation is far less black-and-white than it may appear, however. Those who teach us don't intend to be deceptive. For the most part, physicians are outstanding human beings with an abiding love of mankind and a true interest in improving the world. But somewhere on the path of medical education that we all tread, the inconsistencies and irregularities of modern medicine become acceptable faults for which we are asked to compensate, often through neglect or even active repression of our own intellectual curiosities. We deny or repress awareness of the gaping fault lines that we had at one point questioned, and we accept the silence or evasion that met our first innocent questions. Now we're in the awkward and unfair position of having to repair what was broken before we arrived.

In what is partially a nod to Samuel Shem's timeless and brutally cutting satire *The House of God,* physicians often refer to the modern medical world as the "House of Medicine." My field, emergency medicine, is a specialty that by its very nature straddles the line separating medicine from the rest of society—we're both inside the House and a part of the world outside. If there is a structural analogy, emergency medicine is the porch, or threshold, of the House. Emergency departments tend to be situated at the literal edge of each hospital, functioning as the gateway for the ill and injured. Emergency medicine personnel interact with the outside community but are also deeply integrated with the daily functions of the hospital, its staff, and its culture. The field of emergency medicine is a relative newcomer to the House (it became a recognized medical specialty in 1979), and therefore offers a somewhat new perspective on the establishment. We are constantly challenged in emergency medicine to innovate, to adjust to the unexpected on a moment's notice. Traditions and embedded assumptions are often obstacles to clear thinking, detriments to time-pressured problem solving. Therefore constant reevaluation of our practice, our subculture, and our community is an ongoing daily task. For us, a fresh eye isn't just valuable, it is essential.

Because it is the focus of my experience and because it offers a unique vantage point, I use anecdotes from the emergency department, and occasionally from my experiences in medical school, paramedical work, and the U.S. Army's 344th combat support hospital in Iraq, throughout the book. Emergency medicine is where modern medicine meets the people, and situations from this environment often illustrate, sometimes starkly, the underlying strengths and ills of our system. Other than the changing of names and some identifying circumstances, the scenarios I describe are true.

The essence of medicine is a profoundly human, beautifully flawed, and occasionally triumphant endeavor. These are conditions that must be acknowledged by physicians and laypeople. By no means do I want to dissuade people from seeing their physicians, nor do I want to disrupt their faith in the potential of modern medicine to heal, comfort, and inform. On the contrary, when the truth about medicine is laid bare, fear of it should be vanquished. When the lines of communication are open and the darkest corners are illuminated, we should all be comfortable in the House together. My attempt to shed light is therefore born of a genuine love for the Art. Mine is a field of boundless intellectual challenge, one in which I learn daily not one but many new things; a field in which honest, open interaction nearly always brings mutual benefit. My respect for medicine leads me to believe that our current flaws, deep as they may be, are entirely repairable, and that modern medicine can successfully emerge from the shadows.

SECRETS FROM
THE HOUSE OF MEDICINE

1

WE DON'T KNOW

"*D*r. Newman, phone call, 6800.*"

"*Emergency department, Dr. Newman,*" *I answered,* *thinking the call was likely to be a doctor's office sending me* *another patient on a busy Monday.*

"*T, honey?*" *She used my childhood nickname, as she always does.*

"*Mom?*"

"*Yes, sweetie.*" *She forced the breath between her lips.* "*Honey,* *something's wrong. I need some help.*"

"*What do you mean, Mom?*" *A knot started in my stomach. My* *mother is stoic and selfless, and doesn't ask for help (she doesn't want* to impose). That she was asking for help and "bothering" me at work were both ominous signs.

"It hurts in my stomach, baby. It started a few minutes ago, all of a sudden. I don't know what to do."

"Are you at work, Mom?"

"Yeah."

"I'm calling an ambulance for you. You're going to come here now."

"No, sweetie, thank you, but that's too much drama for the office."

I shook my head. She apparently believed that she could settle gently to the floor like a leaf, passing quietly into the next world, and that this would be preferable to causing a scene.

"Give Heather the phone, Mother."

I spoke to her assistant at the next desk, who was, as I would've guessed, oblivious—not because of inattentiveness but because my mother doesn't complain. Heather escorted her into a cab and brought her to the emergency department. When she arrived, she was doubled over and visibly short of breath. A colleague I trust and respect evaluated her.

My colleague performed a rapid history and physical examination. She had blood drawn for tests, chest and abdominal X-rays, an electrocardiogram, oxygen administered through her nose, a heart monitor, and two intravenous lines placed in her arms—all within the first few minutes. Tests for liver disease, pancreatitis, gallstones, internal bleeding, ulcers, gastritis, and kidney stones were normal. Blood tests and X-rays for her heart and lungs were normal, and she showed no signs of serious infection. She underwent a computed tomography (CAT) scan of her abdomen to evaluate her intestines, her appendix, her aorta, and the rest of her abdominal organs, and we did a bedside ultrasound to see her liver and the blood vessels in her abdomen. All of these were normal. And slowly she began to feel better, with no particular treatment.

After three hours of observation and a battery of test results, the colleague I had handpicked to see my mother shrugged sheepishly, apol-

ogized, and said, "I don't know, I just don't know. I'm just gonna call it 'abdominal pain.'"

———————

"Undifferentiated abdominal pain" was my mother's diagnosis. It is a trash-bucket term that means we don't know what caused the problem. It also means we have found no reason to believe it's dangerous (arguably good news), and it's likely, though not guaranteed, to go away without any particular treatment. In other words, we don't know what caused it, we don't know what to do about it, we don't know if it'll come back, and we don't know where to go from here. Undifferentiated abdominal pain could more accurately be called a nondiagnosis.

What's perhaps most remarkable about my mother's experience is how utterly unremarkable it is. Mom got better. As inexplicably as her pain appeared, so too did it disappear. Over the next few days she went for an official ultrasound of her liver and gallbladder, and two follow-up appointments with her physician. The nondiagnosis did not change. Roughly 40 percent of visits to the emergency department for abdominal pain are ultimately categorized as undifferentiated abdominal pain; no definitive diagnosis is made and no successful diagnostic or therapeutic procedure is performed. What's surprising, however, is how rarely doctors say the words "undifferentiated abdominal pain" to the patients who experience the problem. Much more often a provisional, specific diagnosis is given—maybe "peptic ulcer disease," or "ovarian cyst," or "colitis," but when a physician makes one of these diagnoses, it's often based on what we call "clinical criteria." In other words, we take an educated guess, but we don't know.

An extremely common example of a provisional diagnosis is "gastritis," or inflammation of the lining of the stomach. Gastritis is usually associated with nausea, vomiting, and pain, and can be precisely and accurately diagnosed only by looking at the inside of the stomach through a camera. This requires an invasive test called "endoscopy," and we rarely do it in the emergency department (except in extreme, life-threatening situations). Therefore, while gastritis is a common provisional diagnosis in emergency departments and medical offices, the only method to definitively diagnose it is rarely performed in emergency departments or medical offices. And disturbingly, studies have shown that when physicians think the problem is gastritis, they are frequently wrong.*

Abdominal pain is only one example from a long list of symptoms or conditions that, despite its advances, modern medical science cannot diagnose or explain. Do you know what causes the sound of knuckles cracking? No? Nor do I. Ask an orthopedist or a dedicated hand surgeon or a rheumatologist and you may get three different answers. In order to determine the mechanism of knuckle-cracking sounds, the House of Medicine has launched meticulous studies, including one that uses minimicrophones to document and gauge the amplitude and decibel level of the sounds produced. But we have no definitive answer. Do you know what causes memory loss or unconsciousness when a concussion occurs? Neither do we. Do you know what a concussion actually is, at a biological or cellular level? Me either. Do you know what epilepsy is, or what causes the seizures that characterize this condition? Ditto. The list goes on and on. While we can cure some previously fatal cancers, rid the

---

*A review of studies assessing physicians' (specialists' and primary care physicians') ability to diagnose gastritis and ulcers without endoscopy recently concluded that "symptoms appear inefficient for diagnosing the presence or absence of disease." In other words, without endoscopy, physicians are highly inaccurate at diagnosing the disease.[1]

world of scourges like smallpox and polio, and map the human genome, we don't know what makes a knuckle crack.

Comprehending the cracking of a knuckle may seem relatively unimportant, but as a symbol of the vast and uncharted range of biomedical science, it's not trivial at all. Grasping the limits of physician knowledge is critical to deriving a benefit from medical care. Unfortunately, physicians often *act* as though they know all the answers, and patients often *presume* that physicians know them, when in fact physicians do not. This combination of unconscious prevarication and mutual misunderstanding is one of the wedges that has forced open the chasm between doctors and patients. As a result of this dysfunctional paradigm, when a diagnosis, or even a cause for a diagnosis, is unknown—an entirely common and reasonable occurrence, given the state of our science—people become angry. And in America, anger is often followed by lawsuits.

An example of this, one that is not unique but that garnered an unusual level of popular media coverage, is the story of silicone breast implants and the legal actions and FDA proceedings that followed. Contrary to the number of successful lawsuits that have convinced juries of a link between silicone breast implants and lupus (and other, similar diseases), the research on this supposed link is fairly conclusive: the incidence of lupus among women who've had silicone breast implants is the same as the incidence of lupus among women who haven't had breast implants.[2] Any woman can develop lupus, including those with silicone breast implants, but the two are not related.

Difficult as it may be to understand for frustrated women who develop lupus shortly after getting implants, it is a fact. Lupus is a poorly understood disease of the human immune system that can cause rashes, joint pains, kidney disease, and other serious problems, and while it's not very common, it occurs frequently in women in their twenties and thirties, the same age at which many women obtain breast implants. By random chance alone, then, there was bound to be crossover between these two populations—but no association has been established. Unfortunately, however, while we seem to have ruled out silicone breast implants as a cause, we don't know what *does* cause lupus—or rheumatoid arthritis, or scleroderma, or the other autoimmune diseases that misguided lawsuits have claimed were related to silicone implants. If we did know the cause, then the frustration of coping with these diseases would be channeled into a cure, and any effort to hold silicone responsible for lupus would be less likely to find support in a courtroom or anywhere else.

The bottom line with lupus, with knuckle cracking, and with much abdominal pain is that we don't know what causes them, and we don't know what to do about it. Given the blistering pace of biomedical advances and technology, one would think that our biomedical knowledge would grow every day, and in some ways it does. But this immense "we don't know" category also grows every day.

Erica shrugged. "I know, I can't believe it either." The physician ID tag clipped to her belt with a photo of Erica's enthusiastic smile seemed out of place, a glib reminder of how quickly life can turn.

Ian shook his head in disbelief while Mark, Cary, and I stared at Erica, confused. "Multiple sclerosis? You're kidding. Wow. Blurriness? That was it? Wow." Ian had never been accused of eloquence, but he was voicing what all four of us were thinking. As residency classmates the four of us had grown close, and Erica was one of the brightest, best doctors I've ever known. She had just been diagnosed with MS.

I tried to understand it. "How? I mean, from what?"

"That's what I wanted to know," Erica said. "But who knows,

man, who knows?" She threw her hands up. "I've read about it a lot, but it's like an X-file, this freaking thing. You wouldn't believe it."

"What are you gonna do?" I asked. We were all wondering. We wanted to hear that she would stay a part of our lives. "Can we do anything?"

"Nah, it's chilled out a lot. I feel okay. I think I'm just gonna keep on. It's crazy, huh?"

I breathed a small sigh of relief, but my classmates and I never really came down from it. Two years later I saw Erica at a medical conference and she looked radiant, with her athletic frame and her beautiful smile. And I still wondered—how, from what? How could this be?

Multiple sclerosis is a prime example of medicine's rudimentary understanding of disease, a condition characterized by the dysfunction of nerves in the brain and body due to the degradation of their outer lining. As with many diseases that involve gradual loss of function in the nervous system, the cause is unknown and there is currently no cure. The classic medical school teaching about MS is that it is a condition "disseminated in time and space," meaning it's both temporally intermittent and symptomatically diverse—it affects patients at different times in their lives, and also in different locations of their nervous system. MS typically develops slowly, exhibiting oddly disparate and changing symptoms, and so can be difficult to diagnose. The symptoms range from the mild, such as tingling of an arm, to the severe, including paralysis or loss of coordination. While many people with the disease live a long and somewhat uneventful (in terms of MS) life, some do not. Most individuals experience either mild symptoms or moderate to severe episodes periodically, but a small group experiences an unpredictable, progressive, and occasionally fatal deterioration.

While it's disturbing that we haven't yet established a prognostic marker, a cause, or a cure for MS, what really perplexes scientists is the strange set of patterns they've discovered in who contracts the disease. My colleague Erica was born near Bennington, Vermont, a quiet and beautiful New England town that like many other towns in the northern United States has become a virtual flash point for MS.

Why does Bennington have one of the highest MS rates in the world? We don't know, but we can read the maps that show it to be true. Studies of epidemiologic trends have established that the highest incidence of MS rests firmly at this latitude, 40 degrees or greater, throughout much of the industrialized world. If you're born in northern Wisconsin, or in the Scottish Highlands, or in New Zealand at latitude that's 40 degrees or more from the equator, your likelihood of developing MS is strikingly similar to that of people born in Bennington, Vermont.[3]

The apparent consistency of this geographic mystery has been illustrated in studies time and time again. As if to prove that it's not a statistical anomaly or fluke, the incidence of MS also decreases consistently and incrementally as one's birthplace moves toward the equator. If Erica had been born in Florida instead of Vermont, her chance of developing MS would've been only one-quarter of what it was. However, had she been born in the state of Washington or Wisconsin (both about the same distance from the equator as Vermont), it would've been virtually the same.

Even stranger, had Erica moved to Florida as a young child she would've assimilated with the locals. That is to say, her chance of developing MS would've become roughly the same as that of those born in Florida. But if she had moved to Florida after adolescence (roughly age 15), her chance of developing MS would've remained the same as if she had never moved.

The epidemiology of MS is, as Erica said, a medical X-file, a total mystery. Potential geographic and atmospheric triggers—including environmental toxins, intensity and duration of sunlight exposure, temperate viral and bacterial infections, temperature and humidity changes, diet, electromagnetic differences, and more—have all been studied exhaustively. None of these factors appears to be independently associated with MS. In fact, new questions often arise from such studies. One finding is a strange exception to the latitude rule: for Alaskan native Inuits, regardless of latitude, diagnoses of MS are almost unheard of, or are at least extremely rare. There's no reasonable explanation for this, either.

As interesting and strange as these idiosyncrasies in the geography of MS may seem, the point that they illustrate is clearly more than a novelty. Erica was born in the northeastern portion of the United States, and I can assure you that every one of her physician friends has researched this mystery with a deep personal curiosity and a wish to discover something helpful or important, yet we could not, nor could the numerous other physicians or scientists devoting their time and work to this phenomenon. We remain hopelessly ignorant about why people get MS, and one product of our ignorance is that the only treatments for the disease are poorly developed and nonspecific.

While this epidemiologic puzzle highlights how much we have to learn about the complex disease of MS, there are basic issues encountered every day that perplex us equally. One of the great mysteries of modern medicine is one of our most ubiquitous and seemingly simplest nuisances—back pain.

Sergeant Cole was a gunner normally posted in the turret of a Humvee, an aggressive and watchful sentinel protecting convoys throughout the

Baghdad area for the United States Army. Outside of our emergency department, on dusty streets and forbidden highways, Cole wore sleek black shades and a quiet confidence. Built like a weight lifter and sporting shrapnel scars up and down his right arm, neck, and flank from his first tour in Iraq, the sergeant was admired on the base, known for razor-sharp vision and coolness under fire. As the reigning champion of the widely attended Friday Night Fights on the base, Cole was even something of a celebrity. He inspired knowing nods and crisp salutes from the enlisted, and he carried himself proudly.

Inside our emergency department, however, things were different. Ever since an awkward miss with a left hook in the boxing ring a month earlier, Cole had suffered from gripping back pain and spasms. On this day in late October he limped into the hospital tent squinting in pain, dropped his body armor on the floor, and hoisted himself onto one of the cots. He lay on his side and called weakly to the nurse.

"Ma'am, Major Z, I need a shot. Please."

Major Z looked at me over her glasses, and though it was the third time this week, I nodded. She opened the locked pharmacy box and drew out a syringe with narcotics in it.

"Doc, tell me what to do." Sergeant Cole stared at the side wall of the tent. "It's killing me up there." He was referring to being in the turret, semisquatting and semistanding for hours on end with forty pounds of equipment and protection strapped to his torso.

"Sergeant, your gunner days are over. We talked about this last time: I don't know what's going on in that back of yours, but I know it's time for you to take up something else. Something that won't tear you up or get you addicted to drugs. I'm going to talk to your commanding officer today."

"I went to physical therapy every day like you said. I took the pills you gave me. I did the exercises. Why's nothing working?"

I shook my head. "Don't know, Sergeant."

Cole nodded slowly, and his eyes welled up as the nurse injected his arm with morphine.

Musculoskeletal back pain—pain arising from the muscles and bones of the back—is one of the most common afflictions in the world. It's estimated that 70 percent of humans experience severe back pain at some point in their lives, and in the United States, this results in tens of thousands of surgeries each year. Healthy, fit, athletic people like Sergeant Cole get it as often as those who are physically unfit, but those whose backs and torsos are asked to carry uncommonly heavy loads are at exceptionally high risk.

As common as back pain is, however, physicians and researchers are mystified as to what causes it. At a cellular level, it's an enigma. Is it twisted muscle fibers? Irritated nerves? Involuntary spasms? No one knows. No research has ever taken a microscopic look at the muscle cells and fibers of someone having back pain and then compared them to identical cells and fibers from healthy individuals. Why has no one performed this study? For one thing, it's a tough study to find volunteers for—we'd have to excise a chunk of their muscle to get the cells and fibers. For another, such a study may not even give us an answer.

What about using magnetic resonance imaging (MRI) to detect the cause of back pain? MRI, which is noninvasive and shows major muscle changes fairly well, continues to be the test of choice to evaluate back pain—particularly to detect causes that are *not* muscular in origin, such as nerve compression and spinal cord problems. But there's a secret about MRIs and back pain: the most common problems physicians see on MRI and attribute to back pain—herniated, ruptured, and bulging discs—are seen almost as commonly on MRIs of healthy people without back pain.* This means that herniated and bulging discs, and most of the other findings that radiologists report seeing on MRIs of the back, usually have nothing to do with back pain.

There are exceptions, of course,† but herniated discs on an MRI most often are not an indication of a problem. They are a normal finding, suggesting that discs (the cartilage that cushions the area between the back bones) rupture, or herniate, with some frequency, and our bodies repair them uneventfully. Surgery to fix or remove a disc is usually performed in the hope that a herniated disc is compressing a nerve and causing the pain, but it carries a poor overall success rate. Even after the nerve is "decompressed," or freed, by removing the disc surgically, half of the time the patient's low back pain is unrelieved.‡ This is likely because disc rupture and natural repair is common, an explanation that calls into question the widespread use of back surgery for ruptured discs. When I was in medical school a neurosurgeon once told me he didn't believe in back surgery. Given that we

---

*The range of herniated discs in normal healthy people is 20–76 percent, while the range for bulging discs is 20–81 percent.[4]

†When a colleague during residency twisted his back playing golf and within a few hours was dragging his left foot behind him, an MRI showed a herniated disc pressing on the nerve area that controls his left foot. An emergency operation brought some function back to his foot, though slowly and incompletely. In this case the ruptured disc was pressing firmly enough on the nerve that the nerve began to die. And in general when the results of an MRI demonstrate exactly the problem that a patient's symptoms suggest, in exactly the expected location, and particularly when there is muscle weakness (this is rare), a herniated disc is a likely cause for the problem.

‡This is a controversial point. It has been widely suggested by back surgeons that poor selection of patients is the reason for most surgery failures. The cure rate from large studies ranges from 58 to 93 percent.[5] However, in trials and series assessing long-term results, outcomes are generally unfavorable: one-third to one-half of patients report being unsatisfied, while a moderate percentage experience some short-term, but no long-term, benefit to surgery.[6] A recent, large-scale randomized trial was, predictably, able to find no meaningful differences between those who do and do not have surgery for the same back pain problems.[7]

were scrubbing and prepping for a back surgery that he was about to perform, I found this slightly disconcerting. I asked why we were doing the surgery. He shrugged. "It's good practice."

The result of our ignorance about the actual pathology of back pain is that we have no cure for it. We can treat it with pain medicines, and we do, and they are temporarily effective. But we give people who have severe or chronic back pain the same medicine that we give to those who have knee or pancreas pain, or even cancer. And treating the pain doesn't mean that in a few days, weeks, months, or even hours, the pain won't come back. It usually does. Therefore Sergeant Cole suffered, and eventually had to give up his boxing and his gunning, because we were unable to help him. The existence of countless alternative fields that thrive on the treatment of back pain, including chiropractic medicine, acupuncture, and massage therapy, is due to medicine's failure to help back pain sufferers. Where alternative and complementary medicine has flourished, it's nearly always a sign of modern allopathic medicine's failure, and back pain is the prototype. While many well-intentioned, reputable, and effective physicians prescribe treatments or perform surgeries for back pain every day, the honest truth is that back pain is fraught with we-don't-know.

In his teachings to neophyte practitioners and students, Hippocrates cautioned physicians to "make no pretense to infallibility." As one might expect of a physician practicing in an age before the accurate elucidation of human function and disease, he was acutely aware of his lack of knowledge. Given this lack, his success as a physician and a physician-educator is mystifying. Despite subscribing to the "humors" theory of human health, despite knowing neither the location nor the function of the human heart, and despite being unaware of staple concepts like oxygen or the passage of blood through arteries and veins, Hippocrates was heralded as a man of medical science whom his patients and students loved, and whom the Western world lionized. How can someone with little to no true scientific knowledge still be seen as the great master of medical science?

There's a linguistic clue that may help to explain how a prescientific Hippocrates flourished in, and eventually led, the field of medicine. Those who've attempted to translate the Hippocratic writings for modern readers have often noted an idiosyncrasy in the language: the ancient Greeks made no distinction between "art" and "science." In *Hippocrates,* translator W. H. S. Jones notes in an introductory passage, "The word τέχνη can mean either 'art' or 'science,' though it inclines more towards the former." Discussing the evolution of ancient Greek language, he continues, "We have to wait until Aristotle . . . before there is a word approximately equivalent to our 'science' without any additional notion of 'art.'"[8]

Hippocrates and his contemporaries believed the worlds of poetry, music, and medicine to be fundamentally intertwined. For ancient Greeks the scientist was philosopher and vice versa, as they envisioned their disciplines in a vastly different way than we envision our scientific models of thought and knowledge today. Hippocrates did not see the field of medicine as a storage bin of ultimately knowable facts and figures, and therefore he neither pretended nor aspired to be all-knowing. Instead, he knew his patients.

That doctors often don't have the answers they and their patients seek is a medical secret, the symptom of a quiet and pervasive deception. Physicians are frequently portrayed in popular media as all-knowing, and are often looked to for answers or expertise far beyond the reaches of our limited science and our narrow training. And yet a physician friend once told me that he learned during medical school that there are two things a doctor never says: "I don't know" and "I was wrong." That is a decidedly un-Hippocratic lesson. Peer behaviors, the examples of our mentors, and the general culture of medicine have all served to reinforce this lesson.

The public's misplaced faith that we have answers to all or even most questions may be flattering, but it has also been quietly corrosive. It takes a grounded understanding of medicine's limits to understand the true healing potential of a visit to the House of Medicine. Recognizing that we're incapable of curing or even understanding many conditions may allow patients to reclaim domain and personal control over their wellness, their illness, and their bodies.

The patient's abdication to the forces of modern medicine and technology is often undertaken with a false impression that there is high potential for cure, or that his physicians possess a detailed understanding of the pathways of his ailment. The truth is that in many cases, given the limits of our science, we don't. This reality only highlights the importance of patient opinions, views, and desires. Physicians are only, after all, consultants to the health of others. What we offer is our consultation and our limited expertise, in the hope that we can collaborate, that we can build a partnership. I tell friends that when a doctor says, "I don't know," it is rarely a sign of weakness or ignorance. More often it's a sign of a physician who knows and appreciates the limits of our science and is willing to be a partner. It's an olive branch of commiseration about what is not, and a hopeful readiness for what is.

2

IT DOESN'T WORK

The paramedics roll the stretcher toward us through the sliding glass doors, and the bouncing soles of bare feet peeking out from beneath a sheet catch my eye. We're in the resuscitation room, waiting. There was an almost unsettling ease in the way the staff chattered casually while preparing the oxygen, opening the code cart, and setting up the heart monitor before the paramedics' arrival. Now they're all business, silent and professional in their crisp movements. The paramedics begin their staccato report ". . . found down . . . shocked . . . pulseless . . . tried everything . . . flatline . . . forty-five minutes . . ." I nod, and I check the heart rhythm while I place a finger on the patient's neck, where a small cross lies. Nothing. We restart CPR, and I notice the cross bouncing.

"Is there family?" I ask.

"They're on the way."

"How far out?"

"Don't know, Doc."

I hold my hands up to the room and shake my head. The nurses record the time. The paramedics shrug and nod. I think to myself that she died forty-five minutes younger than she'll be given credit for. The nurses begin preparing her for her family—cleaning, adjusting, removing.

Tara, the social worker, stands at my side when the woman's sister arrives. The sister shakes her head when I tell her, stomps, begins to scream, and the teenaged daughter cries quietly. I am sorry, so sorry. The family holds the sister as she screams. We bring them to the resuscitation room, where the sister screams louder. No communication is possible. She curses, denounces. She will sue us, she will kill us, she will report us, she will have our license, she will . . . Her son picks her up and carries her toward the exit as she kicks and struggles.

As they pass, the ambulance doors slide open and another pair of bouncing feet catch my eye. The daughter looks at me, still crying quietly, and as I hand her the necklace she tells me that she hopes we don't kill this one too.

Resuscitation attempts for cardiac arrest have become a powerful symbol of modern medicine's success. Dramatic and unlikely recoveries, popularized in film and on television, have captured our imagination, affecting us in ways that may be more global than we understand; the widespread and routine acceptance of CPR and cardiac arrest resuscitation have been accompanied by a societal shift, in which health-care spending in the final year of life (and predominantly the final one to two months of life) now represents nearly a third of our system's total health expenditures.[1] This evolution has been largely unchallenged, as we have quietly accepted that serious illness often requires serious treatment, and that not everyone survives. But there is a fundamental presumption in our acceptance—that the expensive and intensive health-care measures we use, like CPR, actually work.

In his groundbreaking book *Sudden Death and the Myth of CPR*, Stefan Timmermans argues that the peace and dignity that once accompanied our final moments have been surrendered to the driving social force of medicine, a force that was supposed to yield miracles. But contrary to popular belief and media portrayals, these miracles are rare. According to large reviews and major studies, the overall failure rate of cardiopulmonary resuscitation, or CPR, ranges from 93 to 99 percent.* Yet if current trends continue, each one of us and each of our family members will likely be subjected to this invasive medical ritual, including the violent, repeated compression of our chests, the forced inflation of our lungs, the prying open of our mouths, the insertion of large tubes into our tracheas, and the injection of powerful cardiac stimulants. For the great majority of us this will yield nothing other than a disturbing physical aftermath: our ribs will be broken, our hearts will be bruised, and our insides will bleed.

The remarkable failure rate of CPR can be explained best by considering a simple but often ignored fact: CPR is performed only on the dead. We seldom understand that those without breath and without a heartbeat are not near death and they are

---

*From multiple large EMS systems, 93 percent failure.[2] From Ottawa, Canada, a study of more than ten thousand cardiac arrests, 95 percent failure.[3] From New York City, 99 percent failure.[4] More recently presented, currently unpublished data from New York City appear to show a rising success rate in the past ten years, from 1 percent up to about 2 percent.

not on the brink of death, they are dead. Death is, as we know, a generally irreversible condition. For a precious few, however, life after death is possible. Who are these precious few? The answer rests in a strange and oxymoronic fact: those who may benefit from CPR are both healthy and dead. However, the majority of those undergoing CPR are unhealthy and dead. Most of those who experience cardiac arrest do so because they have reached the terminal event in a deadly illness, often cancer, long-standing heart or lung problems, serious infections, kidney failure, or hundreds of other conditions. In these cases cardiac arrest is the culmination of a process that has done too much damage to be reversed by pressing on someone's chest or temporarily breathing for her.

But then there are the rare healthy dead in whom cardiac arrest comes without apparent warning or explanation, not as the result of an existing illness. These individuals have suffered a disease called "sudden cardiac death," most often caused by an electrical storm in the heart known as "ventricular fibrillation," a condition that can develop mysteriously and in seconds. Ventricular fibrillation is a sustained fit of electrical chaos that causes the ventricles, the heart's pumping chambers, to cease all pumping and to quiver uncontrollably (that is, to fibrillate). With fibrillation dominating the heart, the pumping action ceases (even as the quivering continues), blood stops moving through the body, and the patient falls instantly unconscious and pulseless—clinically dead. "Defibrillation," a measured electrical jolt, has the power to stun the heart, stopping all motion and allowing the heart to reset and, potentially, to restart. The electricity is not, as many believe, a "jump start"; it is the opposite: a concerted attempt to electrocute the heart, causing temporary paralysis in the hope that the heart will pick up where it left off before the fibrillation occurred.

Ventricular fibrillation occasionally occurs due to a blocked coronary or pulmonary artery, or because of internal bleeding, but for most patients the event appears to be unexplainable and unaccompanied by active illness—which is precisely why it is often reversible. But how often? Due to its uncommon occurrence (only one or two in every thousand persons experiences sudden cardiac death) and the difficulty in studying such an unpredictable phenomenon, for years cardiac arrest researchers have been able only to guess at the percentage of patients who can be potentially revived. The question remained unanswered for decades, until recently, when the answer came from an unusual location for medical research but a common location for those hoping to be one of a lucky few—the casinos of Las Vegas.

In a remarkable study published in October 2000, Dr. Terence Valenzuela headed a group that trained casino security guards in Las Vegas and surrounding areas to perform CPR and defibrillation.[5] Valenzuela then used the recordings from the casinos' comprehensive network of security cameras to analyze the exact moments of cardiac arrest victims' collapse, the responses of the trained guards, and the use of CPR and defibrillation. The video recordings showed people pulling on slots, throwing chips, or playing cards, and then abruptly falling to the casino floor, seemingly dead. They also showed guards rushing to the victims' sides, beginning CPR, and applying cardiac defibrillator machines. The machines quickly evaluated the heart and, if the heart was fibrillating, delivered a burst of electricity. The guards' rapid response (on average less than three minutes to CPR and less than five minutes to defibrillation) resulted in an unprecedented CPR survival rate: 38 percent. In some cases the speechless, bewildered victims of cardiac arrest awoke, realized where they were, and wanted to continue gambling.

The study's success was due, principally, to two factors. The first was patient selection—most of those in the study were functional, active, relatively healthy people: in the rare category of healthy dead. The second was time—rescuers were at the victims' sides within minutes, while fibrillating hearts were still amenable to defibrillation. These two factors explain the enormous 38 percent success rate, and the study therefore gives us critical information about what does indeed work for the healthy dead suffering from sudden cardiac death. But it also tells us something interesting about what doesn't work. Consider the 62 percent of the healthy dead that died. What was done for them? They too were healthy and functional, and rescuers were at their sides in minutes as well. But either these patients did not respond to defibrillation or else their hearts were not found to be fibrillating. When defibrillation fails or the heart is not fibrillating—conditions that describe not only the majority of the healthy dead but virtually all of the unhealthy dead—what is the treatment?

For the past thirty years, this complicated question has had a simple and universal answer, and this answer gives us an unusual window into what does and what doesn't work, both in resuscitation attempts and in the House of Medicine in general. The answer is "ACLS." In an unusual concentration of educational domain, nurses, doctors, and paramedics throughout the world take a unique course devised and run by the American Heart Association, called Advanced Cardiac Life Support—more commonly, ACLS. The ACLS course instructs how to treat patients who fail to respond to initial electrical shocks and those whose hearts aren't fibrillating. The ACLS method includes intravenous fluids, powerful medications, and invasive procedures. Physicians have taught, learned, and implemented the ACLS method with nearly religious zeal for more than thirty years, with a remarkably standardized approach. Professional health-care providers throughout the world treat cardiac arrest using the rote, cookbook-style recipes and flowcharts taught in the ACLS course. But it isn't just the standardization of treatment that's so remarkable; it is that no alternative approach is ever taught, by anyone. The ACLS method is used on more than a million people every year in the United States, and for millions more around the world.* This is notable in light of a vast body of evidence that all leads to the same conclusion: it doesn't work.

Other than those receiving rapid defibrillation, virtually everyone in cardiac arrest dies. In Las Vegas, only those with ventricular fibrillation, and who therefore received rapid defibrillation, survived. That was the only treatment that worked. Everyone else received ACLS treatments, and they died. You will recall that these are healthy dead patients who have rescuers at their sides within minutes—individuals who comprise a group that is by far the most likely to survive. And yet they are no better off than the unhealthy dead. Other studies seem to agree. In 2004 a Canadian group of researchers published a provocative study of more than ten thousand subjects treated for cardiac arrest after a new ACLS-based system was implemented for their ambulance personnel. For years prior to this, the emergency care providers in their system used CPR and defibrillation as their only treatments. In the new system, whenever initial attempts at defibrillation failed or the heart was found not to be fibrillating (the majority of their patients), ACLS treatments—including intravenous fluids, drugs, and other procedures—were aggres-

*Cardiac arrest that is treated by emergency medical service providers is estimated to occur up to five hundred thousand times per year in the United States, and significantly more occur every day inside of hospitals.

sively and rapidly begun. The study compared the survival rate from cardiac arrests in the years before the implementation of the ACLS program to the survival rate in the years after the program began. The result: performing ACLS was the same as doing nothing at all—survival rates were exactly the same both before and after ACLS was added to CPR and defibrillation.*

Physicians have known for years that ACLS treatments don't work. And yet the protocol taught and recommended by ACLS is exactly what most physicians and paramedics have done and continue to do for millions of cardiac arrest patients throughout the world every day. Rather than thinking, attempting new or innovative or even marginally different treatments, we give the ACLS-recommended drugs, we perform the ACLS-recommended procedures, and, at the ACLS-recommended time, we declare people dead. And our research tells us that everything we have just done is an unnecessary ceremony and a proven failure.

The American Heart Association leaders who teach ACLS are very clear about its purpose: to give health-care providers a system, one possible approach, to treating cardiac arrest. The ACLS course materials, the website, and all of its textbooks explicitly say that this is only a suggestion, and that cardiac arrest may be treated in many different ways. But a culture of conformity, inertia, and malpractice paranoia seems to have left physicians and emergency personnel feeling hamstrung, incapable of attempting to do something—anything—different. With full knowledge and ample evidence that it doesn't work, we do it anyway.

---

*In this trial more than ten thousand cardiac arrests were examined while an EMS system developed over an eight-year time period from basic capabilities and equipment (defibrillation, CPR, artificial respiration) to ACLS capabilities (IVs, drugs, etc.). Those who received basic CPR did just as well as those who got ACLS treatment.[6]

There are, in the final analysis, two types of dead people. The unhealthy dead are the ones on whom we unfortunately spend the majority of our resources and time. These individuals are most often identifiable. They are ill and have been ill for some time. CPR is neither humane nor fruitful in such cases. The healthy dead, however, are potentially viable. A small, fortunate group of these will undergo immediate CPR and will then receive rapid and successful defibrillation. For the rest, while there may be treatments that will work, as yet undiscovered treatments that indeed may resurrect these healthy dead, we do not experiment, we do not innovate, and we do not deviate. We seem oddly dedicated to doing what we know will not work.

Unfortunately, cardiac arrest isn't the only affliction for which a standard, common intervention is a proven failure—such cases are peppered throughout the world of medicine. And in some of them it's not just doctors and the public who have endorsed and supported a useless health-care measure. Sometimes it's a third party, and the motivation is an old-fashioned one.

It was 3 A.M. when six-year-old Stevie arrived in the emergency department, trailed by his mom. He had tears in his eyes, and mom had dark circles under hers.

"He won't sleep," she sighed. "He's screaming and holding his ear. We've been through this. It's an ear infection. He needs antibiotics."

"Gotcha." I nodded. Curious about his nickname, I asked Stevie if he knew any Stevie Wonder songs. His mom smiled, and he looked at me like I was crazy and told me he knew them all. To prove it he sang "Signed, Sealed, Delivered" while I examined him, though he cupped his left ear the whole time.

After looking in his ears I said, "You're right, it's an ear infection." I took a small vial with a dropper from my pocket. "And I believe I have just the thing."

Mom looked at me suspiciously. "We want the antibiotic pills," she said firmly.

"This is a pretty effective medicine. It numbs the eardrum and can take away the pain, and antibiotics don't really help with that. In fact, once you get the pain under control, the infection usually takes care of itself. How about we give it a try? It might even mean that everyone could get some sleep."

She was unsure, but she liked the idea of sleep. Stevie lay on his side as I placed a few drops in his ear. After he sat back up, I asked him about a personal favorite. "You know 'Sir Duke?'"

He nodded, smiled, and started singing. "Music is a world within itself . . ." He wasn't cupping his ear anymore.

Mom looked at me, then back at Stevie smiling and singing, then again at me. She eyed me as if I had cheated. "It's that quick?" she asked. I nodded.

Her eyes were wide. "Can I get some of that?" she said.

"You can have the whole thing. And I'll be here two days from now. Come see me if he's not all better. If he is all better, just be sure he sees his doctor next week."

Mom nodded, and smiled ear to ear. Then she began to sing along.

Known in medical circles as an upper respiratory infection (URI), the common cold and its related illnesses, such as ear infections, account for the most patient visits to doctors' offices in the United States. And what is modern medical science's treatment of choice for the common cold? Most people know— sympathy, and whatever treatments might help the symptoms (like the topical pain medicine I gave Stevie). That's about all we have to offer because we certainly don't have a cure. Upper respiratory infections are caused by a large group of heterogeneous viruses, but we have no medications that function effectively against them. If we know that URIs are caused by viruses, why are 50 percent of the patients seen for a URI in this country prescribed antibiotics, which don't work against viruses?

Antibiotics, active in either killing bacteria or in stopping their growth, brought about a revolution in modern medicine in the twentieth century, and laypeople like Stevie's mother tend to be abstractly aware of this. Many patients accustomed to being given antibiotics for minor illnesses now arrive at the doctor's office believing they "need antibiotics." As a general rule, laypeople often don't know which categories of infections are likely to be bacterial and which are probably viral, much less that antibiotics don't treat viral infections—but physicians do. So, for instance, it's extremely puzzling that in the case of throat infections—which are viral more than 95 percent of the time[7]—patients and physicians alike tend to think first of the bacterial "strep" infection ("strep" is short for the bacteria *Streptococcus pyogenes*) when sore throat strikes. The result is that more than 70 percent of adults with sore throats are prescribed antibiotics.

The same trend holds for bronchitis, an infection affecting the upper portions of the lung passages. Many studies and large reviews have compared antibiotics to placebos for acute bronchitis and concluded that antibiotics are unnecessary and offer no significant benefit.[8] In addition, antibiotics have a significant downside: they produce common side effects such as diarrhea, allergic reactions, rashes, and yeast infections, as well as rarer side effects such as fatal or nearly fatal allergic reactions, liver problems, and severe skin reactions. Their extremely frequent administration has also bred an ongoing international crisis of antibiotic resistance. This means that in the aggregate, antibiotics are harmful both in the short and in the long term (when there's well-documented risk and little-to-no benefit, the risk/benefit ratio is an easy calculation—it equals harm). But again, most patients diagnosed with bronchitis are prescribed antibiotics.

It may be surprising to learn that antibiotics don't work for bronchitis, or sore throats, or even colds. The trends in antibiotic use for nonbacterial diseases have been present for decades, during which generations of Americans have come to believe that antibiotics are a necessary treatment for such ailments. People often visit their physician between roughly three and seven days from the beginning of their symptoms, and the average viral illness lasts approximately seven to ten days. In most cases, then, the illness is about to abate regardless of whether or not antibiotics are taken. But patient belief in the power of antibiotics is reinforced by the coincidence of their feeling better just days, or even hours, after the first antibiotic dose.

As unseemly as it might appear, a patient's open desire for antibiotics can be very persuasive to a doctor—particularly in a for-profit medical world where patients vote with their patronage for the physician (and sometimes the health plan) they like best.* That consideration aside, from the physician perspective prescribing antibiotics is simple and convenient. Physician time pressures are immense, and the brief encounter with a patient that includes only a look in the back of the throat and a prescription for antibiotics can often feel like a mutually beneficial moment. The physician is out the door and the patient is pleased with what seems like a curative treatment.

There is, however, real danger in this approach. If it's conservatively presumed that 95 percent of antibiotic prescriptions for

---

*See chapter 7, "Meaning Is Missing," for an additional dimension to this problem.

sore throat are unnecessary, then the number of "unnecessary" allergic reactions can be calculated. In the most recent estimate, approximately 13.5 million sore-throat visits were logged to U.S. outpatient providers and emergency departments in 2002.[9] We know that approximately 72 percent of these visits result in a prescription for antibiotics. This means an estimated 9.2 million unnecessary prescriptions for sore throat.* It has been further estimated that life-threatening allergic reactions to amoxicillin, a common and inexpensive antibiotic, occur one out of every 410 times it's administered.[10] Presuming hypothetically that all of the prescriptions were for amoxicillin (an antibiotic considered comparatively safe), one could expect roughly twenty-four thousand life-threatening allergic reactions each year from the unnecessary antibiotics. Giving antibiotics for viral disease is essentially a large-scale game of Russian roulette, and there are thousands of losers.

Physicians have made routine some practices that are openly ineffective, and patients have unknowingly encouraged and fostered this trend. But there's a third group involved as well, one that provides some of the most effective contributions to this campaign of fruitless and potentially dangerous therapies. It is the most goal-directed group in the mix: the pharmaceutical companies.

As we have said, the estimated 13.5 million yearly doctor visits for sore throat result in antibiotic prescriptions 72 percent of the time, which means more than 9.7 million total antibiotic prescriptions—perhaps azithromycin or amoxicillin, or amoxicillin/clavulanate, among others. Amoxicillin, the least expen-

---

*We are presuming for this example that approximately 95 percent of prescriptions are considered "unnecessary." 13.5 million x 0.72 x 0.95 = 9.2 million unnecessary prescriptions.

sive of the three mentioned, costs about $8 for a week's supply, for a potential $78 million in annual sales from sore throat alone. The most expensive is amoxicillin/clavulanate, at nearly $100 for a prescription, for which 9.7 million prescriptions would represent $1 billion.

The result of this massive financial potential is, unsurprisingly, relentless and insidious advertising. In one distinctly pioneering example of just how ambitious these campaigns can be, advertisements for antibiotics were directed at small children. Max the Zebra, a creation of Pfizer Inc., was devised to help sell azithromycin (trade name Zithromax). In 1999 and 2000, Pfizer representatives handed out Max, a small plastic zebra, to thousands of pediatricians in an effort to entice them to use the toys to console or entertain ill children. The small plastic Max attaches to stethoscopes, while a soft, stuffed version of Max was handed to physicians to give out to children. Pfizer also sponsored a season of *Sesame Street*, utilized famous *Sesame Street* characters in logo-marked campaigns of educational topics ("Elmo Goes to the Doctor" and "Your Amazing Body with Bert and Ernie"), and even donated a real zebra to the San Francisco Zoo.[11]

Max and his related campaign maneuvers followed on the heels of a highly unfavorable 1999 declaration by the Agency for Healthcare Research and Quality, a branch of the National Institutes of Health, that said that many of the newer, more expensive antibiotics appear to be no better for many types of infections, including ear infections, than older, less expensive ones.* While Pfizer's sketchy timing and dubious use of direct advertising to children were noted by a small handful of popu-

---

*While the AHRQ study did not specifically examine azithromycin, it was widely perceived as attacking all of the new, more expensive antibiotics, azithromycin included.[12]

lar press outlets, an additional fact in the agency's report was missed by almost everyone: the great majority of ear infections will improve without any antibiotics at all.[13]

When a therapy that doesn't work is common and pervasive, it's because physicians, patients, and third parties have all played a role. This three-pronged problem has been around longer than antibiotics and longer than prescriptions; any number of seemingly mundane medical nuisances and their corresponding "remedies" can tell the same old story that colds and antibiotics now tell. Coughing, for instance. Cough is present in bronchitis, URIs, pulmonary diseases, allergies, postnasal drip, sinusitis, the side effects of common blood pressure medicines, and more—the list of common ailments and conditions that include cough goes on and on.

Accordingly, there are countless cough remedies on the market today, typically used by those with infections like bronchitis and colds, both over-the-counter and prescription. There are drops, candies, syrups, lozenges, solutions, powders, pills, "pearls," and lots more. Which works best? Take your pick, because for these infections the most recent research shows none of them consistently works any better than a placebo, and none ever has.* Cough is just one more ailment for which we have no cure, and no effective treatment.

---

*Two large-scale reviews have addressed the question of placebo versus over-the-counter cough medicines, one for children and one for adults. Neither identified a cough medicine that works reliably.[14] The most common prescription cough medicines, including codeine, are equally ineffective.[15] In addition, in 2006 the American College of Chest Physicians released guidelines discouraging use of over-the-counter cough syrups because of a lack of proven effectiveness, and case reports of harmful effects. Not surprisingly, the Consumer Healthcare Products Association, a trade group for makers of over-the-counter medications, disputed the guidelines, as did the makers of Robitussin, one of the top-selling over-the-counter cough syrups.

There is an important point about the power of placebo here—see chapter 7.

That's not to say, however, that physicians don't recommend or prescribe cough medicines. It seems that the triumvirate of patient–medical establishment–corporation exists codependently, with each partner having done its part over time, adding on until a treatment becomes standard, common, and expected. The title line on one Wyeth Consumer Healthcare website reads, "Robitussin. Recommended by Doctors,"[16] while a second site proudly reports the product to be "specially formulated with a proven cough suppressant."[17] No references are given for either of these statements, though while the second is dubious, the first is frequently true. Physicians often do suggest treatment with over-the-counter cough medicine, which we know from studies doesn't work. And when our patients return because it didn't work, many doctors will then order prescription cough medicines, which are proven to be equally ineffective.

The everyday use and endorsement of health-care interventions that don't work is present in many of the personal interactions between doctors and their patients, but the doctor's office is not the only place where this occurs. Large-scale public health measures have also occasionally been subject to political and cultural influences that are nonmedical and nonscientific.

Beatrice shivered as she spoke. "I was afraid. My doctor told me to have it checked last summer, a year ago, but I was afraid. And the mammogram was normal." She looked at the ceiling, trying to ignore me as I began to peel away the blood-soaked left side of her thin, flowered dress. "I just hoped and prayed it was nothing."

"Told you to have what checked?" I asked. Beatrice had been brought in by paramedics who found her on the floor of her retirement-community apartment, too weak to get up and frantically call-

ing for help. She wouldn't allow the paramedics to see under her dress.

She shook her head, and her voice cracked. "Thirty years at the university, and I do something stupid like this."

A medical student gently patted Beatrice's shoulder. "Don't worry, ma'am, I'm sure we can help you get through this, whatever it is."

"Ma'am, what did your physician tell you to—" I stopped speaking when I removed the final undergarment from the left side of her chest, and there was no longer any need for questions. The nurse who had been helping me stepped backward quickly, dropping the IV equipment, and the medical student let out a sound as if she had been punched in the stomach.

Beatrice's left breast was largely gone, replaced by a yellow-red, hard, lumpy tumor that was eroding through the skin. Pus and straw-colored fluid ran in slow rivulets across the tumor's surface, and blood oozed from an area where the cancer had recently broken through. I used gauze to hold pressure there, though fly larvae were clustered in the area and crawled about, obscuring the source of the blood.

"Oh, dear. I'm so sorry." Beatrice held one hand to her mouth as she grasped the medical student's hand with the other.

Beatrice had a mammogram just weeks before she found a lump in her left breast, and that mammogram had been read as normal. She rationalized, allowing her fear of doctors and the results of the mammogram to profoundly color her judgment, and within months the lump had grown through her skin. For many women like Beatrice, mammograms are their primary means of breast cancer vigilance, and many women have come to believe in mammograms so strongly that they rely only on them. But how good are mammograms? When breast cancer is present, how often will a mammogram miss it?

The answer for screening mammography is straightforward. Roughly 25 percent or more of cancers are missed. In research studies on mammograms at least one in every four cases of breast cancer is found after a "normal" mammogram. Beatrice's case is an example.* Twenty-five percent may seem like a disappointing number, but it's true nevertheless that 75 percent of cancers will be detected by mammograms. One might argue, therefore, that this makes mammography a useful test. Despite the imperfection, identifying up to three-quarters of breast cancers should be a step in the right direction. But the reality is less clear-cut. As with any test, the most important question is whether or not the benefits outweigh the costs and risks. So before we talk about the benefits of mammograms, what precisely are the costs and risks?

Perhaps the most universal risk of a medical test is the possibility that there will be "false positives," or results that indicate a disease is present when it is not. False-positive mammograms are particularly serious, leading to further testing, unnecessary surgeries, and the considerable anxiety associated with being informed that one may have cancer. So how often do mammograms produce false positives? The cumulative risk of having a false-positive mammogram in ten years is 50 percent; therefore half of women undergoing regular mammograms for ten years will receive a "positive" result that is

---

*This statistic is from *studies* of mammography, in which highly specialized and trained mammogram readers tend to be involved. The number is therefore probably significantly higher (more cancers are missed) outside of research studies. A recent editorial in *The New England Journal of Medicine* claimed, although without any hard evidence, that up to 50 percent of all breast cancers in the United States are first diagnosed after a lump is found, but then subsequently noted to have been visible on the patient's previous mammogram.[18] As reported on in-depth in *The New York Times,* consistency and accuracy in reading mammograms is a serious, and equally controversial, problem.[19]

incorrect. Indeed, 97 percent of "positive" mammograms are false rather than true.* These data help to explain why surgical biopsies on normal breasts occur so frequently. During ten years of mammograms about 20 percent of women, or one in every five, will have a false positive that leads to a biopsy.† Finally, false positives take a psychological toll: half of women who have false-positive mammograms report at least three months of "substantial anxiety."[22]

In addition to anguish, increased surgeries, and further testing, there is the financial cost of mammograms. There are 100 million women over the age of forty-five in the United States, and roughly 70 percent appear to routinely obtain mammograms. Mammograms cost approximately $100 to $150 each, which tallies to about $4 billion spent on mammograms per year, presuming biennial screening. This excludes lost workdays and the peripheral costs such as travel and follow-up visits. Importantly, it also doesn't include the follow-up testing, reimaging, surgeries, and complications that occur just due to false positives, problems that inevitably result in more lost workdays and more procedures (a breast biopsy runs from about $1,000 to $5,000). If 70 million women have mammograms and one in every five has a biopsy due to a false positive, then we can estimate that between $14 billion and $70 billion is spent performing surgical procedures on normal breasts.

A final risk/cost to consider is the risk of actually causing cancer due to radiation from the mammogram. For every 10,000

---

*A false positive is just what it says: a test reading that says that cancer is present (a positive reading) when cancer is not present. Ninety-seven percent of positive mammograms are wrong.[20]

†The cumulative risk of a false positive was 49 percent and the cumulative risk of a biopsy for a false positive was 19 percent.[21]

women screened routinely over ten years, it has been estimated that one case of breast cancer is caused by the radiation. With 70 million women in the United States undergoing routine mammograms, we can estimate that mammograms cause about seven thousand additional cases of breast cancer for every ten years of screening.[23]

Given these substantial costs and risks, in order to be considered beneficial mammograms should provide an impressive degree of benefit. To quantify the extent of this benefit, in 2001 the Cochrane Collaboration, a multidisciplinary group of scientists that produces what are widely believed to be the most respected and objective reviews in medicine, exhaustively examined the data on mammograms. The review included scrutiny of the seven largest and best studies ever done, including nearly half a million female study subjects from all over the world. The women were enrolled in studies and assigned to one of two groups: routine checkups including regularly scheduled mammograms, and routine checkups only. The women were then followed for over a decade to determine how many died in each group and how many lived. The total magnitude of the benefit was then calculated across all of the studies, and a rather surprising number was found: zero. Having mammograms was of no benefit at all.

The Cochrane group performed hundreds of statistical calculations, examining dozens of patient and study factors. Their first analysis examined only the two studies of highest quality, which included some 130,000 women. The data from these studies showed that overall, after an average of thirteen years of follow-up time, the same number of women were alive in both groups. Next, concerned that they had excluded potentially important data, the group examined the seven largest studies, including the five they had previously excluded due to problems with quality. When the data from all seven studies were examined, however, little had changed.* Women were alive and surviving at the same rate whether they had been assigned to receive mammograms or not.

How can this be? How can it be that all major media outlets regularly assert that mammograms save lives? How can physicians routinely recommend mammograms? How can professional medical societies such as the American Medical Association, the American College of Radiology, and the American College of Surgeons all recommend regular screening mammograms? There are complicated, uncomfortable issues raised by these questions.

One answer is that, despite this large study, the subject is still not considered settled by the medical establishment. There were detailed criticisms of the Cochrane analysis,[24] and professional societies have been unwilling to change their long-standing recommendations, preferring to stick with the status quo.

Critics of mammograms, however, have speculated that these professional medical societies may hold the key to widespread use and acceptance of mammograms in the face of such powerful evidence. Professional medical societies like the AMA are where large-scale medical recommendations, and therefore public perceptions, often first take hold.

We have long ignored an essential fact about professional medical societies like the AMA: they are advocacy groups. The AMA exists to advocate for all physicians, the ACR exists to advocate for radiologists, and the ACS exists to advocate for surgeons. The overarching mission of these societies is to provide lobbying and advocacy for their constituents, who pay annual

*See the note at the end of this chapter for a more in-depth look at the results of these trials.

dues. It is not to provide objective factual information to the public, nor to make recommendations for medical care. While it is unlikely that anyone at the AMA, ACR, or ACS would be intentionally disingenuous, the recommendations of these groups routinely embrace a position that will most benefit their constituency.* The recommendation by the ACR to use mammograms, for instance, directly supports the radiology establishment. Mammograms mean big reimbursements, big money, and a large role for radiologists in routine preventive care. In addition, as we have noted, many mammograms are positive, and although 97 percent of these are false, it will take lots of surgical procedures to sort out which ones are and which ones are not. The recommendation for women to undergo routine mammograms also therefore supports the referral of millions of women for surgical procedures. This ultimately means payments for services to both the radiological and surgical establishments.†

The problem of professional-society recommendations is not new. In an attempt to ensure objective, evidence-based recommendations from the professional societies, the Institute of Medicine disseminated standards in the early 1990s for formulating official guidelines. It had been widely noted that professional medical societies were publishing guidelines that, like ACLS

---

*The psychology literature is replete with studies showing that conflicts of interest (money, opinions, favoritism, etc.) often bias decisions unconsciously, and sometimes in ways that are cognitively inaccessible to the decision maker. It therefore takes no malice or intent to produce a biased decision.

†Despite the fact that 97 percent of positive mammograms are not actually breast cancer, all of the work that is done to prove that each of these positives is false will be done by radiologists and surgeons. This means that when research moneys are allocated for research on breast cancer prevention, the radiologists and surgeons will be that much more likely to receive the very large sums of money that are distributed in the form of grants for research.

from the American Heart Association and screening mammograms from the AMA, often became standard practice despite evidence that they were wrong or unfounded. Unfortunately, the Institute of Medicine's attempt to clean up the guidelines failed: a study published in *JAMA* in 1999 showed that less than half of the reviewed guidelines either met or followed the IOM standards.*

The basic facts about mammograms have been obscured, partly by the political weight behind them (federal legislation both protects reimbursement for mammograms and makes access to them legally mandatory), and partly by professional societies, which endorse them. And yet it is difficult to point fingers. What else is a radiologist to do when a woman is referred for a routine mammogram? And what else is a surgeon to do when a mammogram indicates a potentially cancerous area in a woman's breast?

To profoundly understate: the problem is complex. Nonetheless, the best data we have, reviewed by our most respected scientists, tell us that mammograms did not save lives in nearly a half million women in whom they were studied. One reason that this fact is so vexing, so difficult to swallow, is that mammograms should work. The idea of mammograms is reasonable, the logic is sound. If what we understand about cancer is correct, if intervening at an earlier stage of cancer is beneficial, then mammograms make sense. Women who had mammograms should have had their cancers detected sooner and therefore should have lived longer—they should have been less likely to die. But they weren't. Could it be that our premise is wrong?

---

*Some guidelines have improved since 1999, but thousands have not.[25]

Could it be that detecting cancer earlier doesn't always mean saving lives?

Two remarkable studies published in 2002 have given us an unexpected answer to these questions.[26] The studies, one from Quebec and the other from Germany, examined what happened when public health officials began massive screening programs in which they tested the urine of infants for traces of a cancer called "neuroblastoma." Neuroblastoma, frequently found in the first two years of a child's life, is among the most common causes of cancer deaths in young children. Researchers and public health officials theorized that by detecting the tumors earlier, at a stage when the cancers were typically both smaller and less aggressive, fewer children would die.

Just as they had hoped, and just as with mammograms, the officials found that by implementing widespread screening they detected many more cancers. But just as with mammograms, they also found that it didn't save lives. In groups that were not screened, children died from neuroblastomas at exactly the same rates as those in groups that were screened. In fact, the study investigators concluded that they were identifying *too many cancers*—nearly 70 percent of the tumors would likely have gone away or else never been found. But once found, all were treated. And the only three children who died in the screening group all died from treatment: two from complications of surgery and one from chemotherapy. All around the world, neuroblastoma screening programs were shut down.

It is impossible to know precisely why it is that mammograms didn't save or prolong lives. But the story of neuroblastomas offers a plausible theory and a critical lesson: finding cancer earlier may not always be the answer. In the case of breast cancer a large proportion of cancerous lumps, perhaps 25 percent or more, are slow-growing and may therefore never lead to serious danger. But just as we did with neuroblastomas, when we find these tumors we virtually always treat them, because we're unable to tell which ones are dangerous and which aren't. The critical concept that emerged from the neuroblastoma studies is that finding cancer is not, in and of itself, a goal. In our zeal to detect cancer we may well have forgotten the real prize: human life.

We need not be despondent about the alternative to mammograms: regular breast exams, particularly by a professional, may well reduce the chance of a cancer being advanced by the time it's found. And they will surely result in fewer false positives. That regular breast exams are a better screening tool than mammograms is a suggestion that has been made before, convincingly.[27] But what's frustrating about the apparent failure of mammograms is that the idea of them seemed so reasonable. Mammograms represent advanced technology, a look inside the human body. It's hard to believe, then, that a manual breast exam is as good as or better than mammograms. But this was precisely what the studies cited above aimed to assess, and the results are in.

While mammograms have been shown not to work for routine screening, there are other purposes for which mammography may work. For patients with lumps, mammograms may provide useful information. In addition, with genetic testing that shows a high familial risk of breast cancer death, mammograms may be a sensible choice. In addition, perhaps decades from now a new study will show that screening mammography can indeed save lives. The original studies were performed in some cases decades ago, and therefore one may argue that our treatments may have more benefit now (although this argument is a stretch that the current data do not support).* Finally, perhaps for a select few who are willing to accept the considerable harm and the costs that accompany them, routine mammograms are an option with the potential to provide peace of mind. These are, however, individual choices to be made between informed patients and their informed doctors, and for such a conversation to occur we'll first need to talk openly about what does and what doesn't work.

Sherwin Nuland, in his timeless work *Doctors: The Biography of Medicine,* describes Hippocrates' contribution to medicine in this way: "There is a moral law which is universally valid, and it is this moral law that pervades the philosophies of the Hippocratics." The oath that bears Hippocrates' name embodies, and also remains an apt symbol for, the message that is clear in his writings. Physicians must be advocates, placing above all else that which is advantageous to patients. It is the application of this philosophy that builds trust, and the healing bond.

There are certainly physicians who aren't aware of the ineffectiveness of many of the health measures they endorse or utilize. But more common, and perhaps more disturbing, are physicians who knowingly use the interventions and medications that don't work, often because of the immense pressures on them from outside of the doctor-patient bond. Advertising, cultural expectations, and misinformed professional-society recommendations, are powerful sources of faulty information that

---

*We should not get ebullient about this possibility. First, there is no evidence to support it; it's pure conjecture. Second, mammograms have enjoyed unfounded support for decades now, and while this argument may become valid at some point in the future, it obviously was not valid ten to twenty years ago, when these studies were performed and initially reported (and when we continued to use mammograms despite the data). The argument therefore is a facetious one to use now.

often make it difficult for physicians to do what is right. Playing out these fruitless rituals is, however, a grand and erosive deception, and it's a turn away from the universal moral law that Sherwin describes and the Oath invokes.

We want something better for ourselves and for our system, and there is no reason to believe that we cannot achieve it. In the case of cardiac arrest, we should be attempting to resuscitate the healthy dead, not the unhealthy dead. In many instances this is a conspicuous distinction and it is one we should seek out. For the healthy dead, however, after an attempt at defibrillation has failed, we can admit that the techniques and algorithms proposed by Advanced Cardiac Life Support are proven to be worthless. We should confront this failure with aggressive research on treatment regimens that have the potential to work.*

And what about antibiotics for ear infections? There are bacteria all over and throughout our bodies, a normal and necessary state. Taking antibiotics often causes uncomfortable diarrhea or yeast infections precisely because of the eradication of the bacterial flora that our bodies depend upon. Therefore with most infections (virtually all colds, bronchitis, sinusitis, ear infections, flulike illnesses, sore throats, sniffles, and the great majority of coughs and fevers), physicians and laypeople should have the same goal: the alleviation of discomfort, not the eradication of the virus. Our immune system will do this for us; that's why we have it. Even when an infection is bacterial, antibiotics are helpful only if one needs them to either survive, avoid permanent damage, or significantly shorten the course of a disease. And

---

*These cases are very likely *not* hopeless. I firmly believe that there may be a role for treatment in these individuals, but ACLS has had its chance for thirty years, and it has failed. Promising work is being done by many.

while studies suggest that doctors are impacted by their perceptions that patients expect or desire antibiotics, numerous studies have shown that these perceptions are frequently mistaken. A physician's capacity for listening and expressing concern matters far more than any prescription.[28]

Then there is the complicated issue of pharmaceutical companies and advertising, a factor known to impact prescribing behavior and to influence (or even create) patient expectations. In an FDA survey in 2003, 62 percent of physicians reported that direct-to-consumer advertising causes tension between them and their patients, and 94 percent noted that it caused patients to believe that the medications work better than they actually do.[29] Physicians know that direct advertising to consumers is harmful, and recognize that allowing advertising to influence them or their patients is virtually impossible to reconcile with Hippocratic ideals.

As for mammograms, if reality and evidence are to be the primary players in women's health decisions, then politics and a culture of wishful perceptions about the ground-level impact of high technology will have to be overcome. As it stands now, women are neither informed about the results of our best mammogram study data nor presented with a true risk/benefit balance. This is an issue that extends well beyond mammography, into many other fields of medicine and testing. Though common, blood tests for prostate cancer have not been proven to save lives.* Colonoscopy screening for colon cancer is also unproven. While it may seem reasonable particularly for those

---

*The PSA (prostate specific antigen) test that is so commonly done is actually very nonspecific, and most authorities do not routinely recommend using it. Furthermore, there is absolutely no reliable evidence that says it saves lives and there is evidence to show that it causes anxiety and further, more invasive testing.[30]

over age fifty (large-scale studies are in progress now), there are known harms, including colon perforation and severe bleeding. It's therefore still not clear if the benefits will outweigh these risks. CAT scans for lung cancer detection is an emerging example—one preliminary study has suggested there may be a lifesaving benefit, while a second has suggested only that surgeries were unnecessarily increased.*

We will have to watch closely in the coming years as the results of clinical trials of these interventions emerge. These screening tests for cancer are in the nascent stages of evaluation or refinement, and yet many of them have already become ubiquitous. We added routine mammograms to our armamentarium many years ago, and we did it without evidence of benefit. Now we know that it is an expensive, probably harmful fait-accompli that is deeply embedded, and we are paying the price. While the high science and simple logic of these tests may seem enticing, we have discovered the hard way that this is not always the case. Partly because of an implicit trust that the various cogs in the medical machine abide by Hippocratic ideals, and perhaps because of a belief that physicians are acting as a concerned and comprehensive filter, laypeople have been led to the false belief that the medical establishment has endorsed these tests on the basis of affirmative evidence of benefit.

Medicine is predicated on trust. Patients trust that a doctor's recommendation to have regular mammograms is based on

---

*The first study suggested a benefit to early detection, but had no control group—everyone in the study got CAT scans—and came to this conclusion using a statistical projection of what "would have happened" had there been no CAT scans on their patient group.[31] The second study used a similar study design, and found the opposite.[32]

evidence. They trust that we write prescriptions because the medicines we dispense have been shown to help. They trust that resuscitation attempts are based on science. We have misspent this trust, and the distance between doctor and patient has grown. The frustrating irony is that many of us, physicians and patients alike, have been led to believe that resuscitation attempts and antibiotics and mammograms are the tools of good medicine.

In truth, these are examples in which we as a system, and we as individual physicians, should take no pride. Individually, we may do our best to stay true to the Oath, and therefore true to patient advocacy. Yet collectively we can look at what we have helped to create and we can see: it hasn't worked.

DAVID H. NEWMAN

Note on Chapter 2

The controversy about whether or not mammograms save lives can be confusing, therefore I will say this first: when one group of women is assigned to have regular mammograms over many years, and they are compared to an identical group that is assigned to have only clinical breast exams each year, then if mammograms are truly effective and beneficial, the women in the first group should, on average, live longer—they should die less frequently. But they didn't.

The argument (one that has been largely relegated to academic halls and conference rooms) about whether or not mammograms save people from death due to breast cancer is partly semantic and partly statistical. A few of the studies that the Cochrane group reviewed did seem to suggest a small reduction in *breast cancer mortality* in the women who had mammograms (about a 20 percent "relative reduction," or about 0.05 percent "absolute reduction"*). However, the Cochrane group felt that these studies and their results were problematic. First, the studies were judged to be methodologically flawed, so much so that they should not be combined with studies that were of higher quality (and that therefore produced more reliable data). When the Cochrane group included only the studies of highest quality in their analysis (studies that included more than 130,000 subjects, a gargantuan

---

*Over a ten-year period women in the breast-exams-only group died of breast cancer at an overall rate of about 0.25 percent. Those in the mammogram group died at a rate of about 0.2 percent. The difference between the two is .05 percent, and is called the "absolute reduction." But a different, and much more impressive, way of saying this is that deaths were reduced by 20 percent, which is technically true. If we only consider the women who died of breast cancer, we can see that this number, 0.25, was reduced by 20 percent, to 0.20. This is the "relative reduction" and because it always sounds more impressive, it is the terminology favored in advertising.

number), they found that mammograms were associated with no improvement in either the breast cancer death rate or the overall death rate—no benefit at all, no matter how you look at it.

However, the benefit that could be proclaimed when the flawed studies were added into the calculation was in the *breast cancer death rate,* not in the *overall death rate.* This is where it gets tricky. Imagine for a moment that a test was devised to identify heart attacks early. We'll call the test the "HeartSaver." Currently, about 10 percent of people who have heart attacks die from them. Imagine, however, that our new HeartSaver test was perfect at identifying heart attacks very early on. The HeartSaver would allow doctors to see the blood flow to the heart with flawless accuracy and therefore determine the exact nature and location of the heart attack. Imagine that this HeartSaver was able to identify all heart attacks so well that no one ever died from a heart attack again. Now imagine that HeartSaver came with an unfortunate side effect: it caused a massive and fatal stroke in 10 percent of the people it was given to. The good news is that no one ever dies of a heart attack if he has the HeartSaver test. The bad news is that, overall, we haven't saved lives; we've simply traded one cause of death for another. And although different people may die if they're given HeartSaver than those who may die if they're not, the overall math tells us that the test isn't worth it. In aggregate, HeartSaver doesn't save lives and would be considered a failure—no one would advocate its use or use it.

Mammograms are the same as the HeartSaver. If we examine the (flawed and dubious) calculation that seemed to show a reduction in *breast cancer mortality* with mammograms, then we also must notice that there is no reduction in *overall mortality* with mammograms. If there is a reduction in a specific type of death in one group, but no reduction in overall deaths, then this means that mathematically there must be an increase in some other type of death in that group. You cannot reduce death from one disease and still maintain the same exact overall death rate without increasing death from some other problem. Therefore, in the mammogram groups from the studies we're discussing, mammograms may have reduced the *breast cancer mortality*, but they must also have, then, increased the mortality from something else. But from what?

First, it is important to understand that with hundreds of thousands of subjects, it is exceptionally difficult to track all data accurately. The mammogram studies are simply too large for us to be able to reliably track down and accurately identify the exact cause of death in every subject, which means we don't have perfect data on the precise cause of death on many of the subjects. That said, hypothetical examples of causes of death that might be due to mammograms would be serious (ultimately fatal) complications from unnecessary breast biopsies, or deaths from cancers caused by mammogram radiation, or deaths due to chemotherapy or surgery for a cancer that would have gone unnoticed (just as in the children whose neuroblastomas were detected and treated). Another possibility is deaths due to suicides related to depression and anxiety provoked by a false-positive mammogram. The list could go on and on.

There is a second possible explanation to consider for the disparity between *breast cancer mortality* and *overall mortality*, and that is "misclassification" of deaths in the group that had mammograms. If deaths in the mammogram group that were actually caused by breast cancer are mistakenly ascribed to some other cause, then this could make it look as if there were fewer *breast cancer deaths* in this group, when in fact the root cause of their death was breast cancer. Examples of this might be women who died from blood clots caused by their cancer (the cause of death might be listed as the blood clot, rather than the cancer that caused the blood clot), or women who die due to a severe infection after their immune system is crippled by chemotherapy (the cause of death might be listed as the infection rather than the cancer that resulted in chemotherapy). If, for instance, a woman died from bleeding complications during a surgery for her mammogram-detected breast cancer, and if her death was classified as due to "complications from surgery," then her death would not be counted as a breast-cancer-related death, when in fact it was. Therefore any number of deaths that are in truth related to the breast cancer can be misclassified, and in a jiffy, on paper at least, it would appear that there is a "reduction in breast cancer mortality" in the group that had mammograms.

Again, which of these explanations is correct, if any, is unclear from the data that we have, but whatever the correct explanation, the bottom line is undisputed: a half million women were assigned in trials either to receive mammograms or not to, and in the end their chances of dying were the same in both groups. Mammograms didn't work.

3

WE DON'T AGREE

"**D**etective." I saw the caller ID and answered my friend Luke's call on the first ring.

"My complainer is hurting," Luke said. He had recently developed plantar fasciitis, a painful inflammation deep inside the heel of the foot. Luke and I had grown up together and he was now a genuine tough guy, a narcotics detective and a sergeant for the NYPD. I had taken to calling his ailment "complainer" fasciitis, which he thought was funny. Seemed like he didn't get the joke.

"Sorry to hear it. Did you rest it for a week like I told you?"

"My doctor told me to stretch it and use it more, not rest it." Luke enjoyed telling me whenever his doctor disagreed with me.

"Oh. Okay, sounds good. So what do you want?"

"Tell me what to do about the pain."

"Okay, ice it. Fifteen minutes on, fifteen off."

"My doctor told me to put a heating pad on it."

"Good idea," I said. *"Try that."*

"Thanks for the consult, smart guy," Luke said, and hung up. About an hour and a half later the phone rang again: *"Detective."*

This time he used his cop intimidation voice. "It still hurts."

"Are you talking about your Complainer Sally-itis?" I asked.

"What'd you just call me?"

"I'm just surprised it's still hurting," I said.

"Uh-huh. What do you suggest, Doctor?"

"Have you tried elevating it above your heart?"

"Well, no, because my doctor told me to keep it low so that the blood flows to it. Do you guys do this on purpose?"

"Hmm. Sure, okay, keep it below your heart."

"Great, thanks. Any other ideas?"

"Well, I'm all out. Have you tried plain old-fashioned drugs?"

"I'm a narcotics cop. That would be like you turning into a heart attack." He sighed. *"How come you never fight for your suggestions being better than my doctor's?"*

"Doctors never openly disagree; we're afraid of fights," I said.

"And I'm the Sally," he said, and hung up again.

Disagreement among doctors is part of the folklore of academic medicine. The disputed diagnosis, for instance, is the lifeblood of the erudite standoff. In challenging cases, respected elders and hopeful young acolytes crowd the bedside, jostling for position, staring at a patient with a mysterious constellation of signs and symptoms, and listening attentively. The eldest physicians in the room will often pose carefully crafted questions, then perform a comprehensive, narrated physical examination, closely watched by all. The patient is then thanked and the audience retires to the hallway, abuzz. To the barely restrained delight of the self-styled intellects (and the deep dismay of the exhausted residents), a feverish dialogue ensues as department heads and textbook authors argue, volleying diagnoses. Each symptom is deconstructed, championed as the potential key to the diagnosis. A patient's offhand remark ("I got this necklace in Borneo recently") or a seemingly trivial complaint ("Isn't it warm in here?") may potentially bring diagnostic revelation. In such moments, trainees, in a flash of brilliance or a stroke of good fortune, may be discovered like starlets at a Hollywood coffee shop.

Such intellectual tempests comprise the great mythologic glory of diagnostic medicine, but in truth they're a far cry from medicine's common, everyday disagreements. Luke's plantar fasciitis, a small area deep inside his foot, was an inflammatory condition that prevented him from exercising for months. But scholars don't debate back and forth in hallowed halls about cold packs versus heat application for an irritating foot condition. Doctors just disagree, and we keep it to ourselves.

This unspoken conflict is important. In some cases it occurs because one physician is right and one is wrong, but more often it points to an inconsistency or a gap in our science and our education, an area in which interpretation, rather than fact, is what drives our medical practice. We often use euphemisms like "differences in style" or "differing schools of thought" or "alternative approaches." But the secret that's too uncomfortable for doctors to embrace or routinely disclose is that we disagree with a frequency that makes it hard to believe that we were trained in the same science. And it's not just minor issues like heat or cold application over which we disagree. In some cases the issues are far more important.

For two days physicians had believed that Patrick, a fifty-three-year-old homeless man and a "frequent flyer" in our emergency department, had a blood clot in his lung, but scans showed nothing. Blood and stress tests for the heart were normal. His chest pain stymied the doctors, and it was summer—Patrick wanted out. According to a witness, when he was discharged from the hospital he stepped into the urban sunlight, squinted as he looked up at our large building, then fell to the ground motionless. He was rolled into the emergency department with a nurse's aide doing CPR.

"Sounds like an arrhythmia," said a colleague as we began to work on Patrick.

"Or maybe a clot," I said. "But I just admitted him two days ago. You'd think they'd have found it upstairs."

Patrick's internist came down to watch the resuscitation and offer ideas, and though there were early signs of hope, our best efforts failed him, again. The next day an autopsy showed a large patch of dead heart muscle. For two days Patrick had been having a heart attack, and we just missed it.

A heart attack, or "myocardial infarction," is a sudden loss of blood flow due to a clogged artery that supplies blood to the muscle of the heart. In Patrick's case, one of the biggest arteries in the heart had clotted off. When a muscle doesn't receive blood (and therefore oxygen), it begins to die, which often hurts and is therefore associated with chest pain. Heart attacks can be reversed, however, by opening the clogged artery before the muscle dies. But this reversal of fortune can occur only if physicians treat heart attacks promptly, and that depends, of course, on identifying them right away.

Physicians use three common methods to identify heart attacks: First, we rely heavily on signs and symptoms. Second, we look for hallmark patterns on an electrocardiogram (EKG). Finally, we look for evidence with a blood test. Unfortunately, none of these methods is perfect; all can miss a heart attack. The blood test can detect damaged heart muscle and is, therefore, in a sense, the best method of the three. But traces of damaged heart muscle don't leak into the bloodstream until at least a few hours after a heart attack has started; therefore sometimes, in the early stages or when the artery isn't fully blocked, there's no detectable damage at all. Patrick's blood tests, for instance, were normal despite a large clot developing in one of his coronary arteries.

The signs (what physicians see, hear, and feel) and symptoms (what a patient reports) of heart attacks are highly varied, although chest pain is among the most common. But most chest pain is not a heart attack; it's benign pain from the chest muscles or the lungs. This makes some heart attacks extremely tricky to diagnose. In many ways it's like searching for a needle in a haystack, though research tells us that certain symptoms do alter the likelihood of pain being from a heart attack. Pain that radiates from the chest to both arms increases the chance that the pain is from the heart, while pain that feels sharp and stabbing is more often from the muscle or lung. Patrick's pain was a "pressure" in the center of his chest (considered typical for heart pain), and breathing deeply made it worse (considered typical for lung pain, not heart pain); therefore in Patrick's case the signs and symptoms weren't very helpful. Nonetheless, because signs and symptoms can in some cases be very important, eliciting and gathering symptoms is considered a critical part of making a diagnosis. One would hope, therefore, that doctors would generally agree about the presence of signs and symptoms in patients potentially having heart attacks.

One well-designed study asked a group of physicians to each separately examine many patients like Patrick, some having heart attacks and some not. After each examination, the researchers asked the physicians to report whether or not they found seven classic hallmark signs of heart failure that can occur during a heart attack, including an extra heartbeat sound (often referred to as a "gallop"), the engorgement of veins in the neck, and fluid around the ankles. Physicians consistently agreed on the presence of only two of the seven signs.[1]

A second study asked physicians to document the symptoms they believed a patient was reporting. The researchers compared agreement on the patients' symptoms between physicians. But they also checked to see how often the patients' symptoms as reported by the physicians agreed with the symptoms as reported by the patients in a written questionnaire. Physicians were unable to consistently agree with one another on six of the ten symptoms. But more remarkably, they overwhelmingly disagreed (nine out of ten) with the *patient* about which symptoms the patient had.[2]*

Much of this disagreement can't be blamed on physicians. Patients are notoriously inconsistent in how they report or perceive their symptoms, which makes identification even more

---

*Research on agreement is somewhat statistically esoteric. "Kappa" values are a statistic commonly used to calculate agreement. Kappa values take into account that there will always be some agreement, even if by random chance. For instance, guessing whether a coin will fall heads or tails, anyone can be expected to be right roughly 50 percent of the time. Kappa values assess how much *more than 50 percent* correct someone is in this situation. Ironically, labeling Kappa values is also interpretive. The potential interpretations frequently reported in the studies noted above (poor, fair, moderate, good, very good) reflect one common method. I have chosen to describe agreement as being "consistent" when a Kappa value was "good" or better on this scale, but not when it was "moderate" or worse.

problematic. As inconsistent as they may be, physicians must rely on signs and symptoms because blood tests are highly imperfect. The faults of both methods led early-twentieth-century physicians to hail the arrival of the EKG, a method for detecting heart attacks that was believed to be potentially objective and accurate, and led to Willem Einthoven's 1924 Nobel Prize in Medicine. Before long, however, the celebration of the EKG had quieted considerably. Physicians disagreed about it too.

An EKG is an electrical portrait of each heartbeat, and to the untrained eye it looks like a piece of graph paper with squiggly lines. While all physicians learn the basic skill of interpreting EKGs, cardiologists, with at least three extra years of training and experience in EKG reading, are considered medicine's experts in the field. But when, in 1958, researchers examined EKG interpretations by ten physicians all experienced in cardiology, the results were surprising. When the ten physicians each read the same one hundred EKGs, they disagreed with one another on the diagnosis two-thirds of the time. In addition, when the cardiologists were secretly given the same EKG multiple times, they also disagreed with themselves more than 10 percent of the time.[3]

With the development of scientific methods and a more nuanced understanding of cardiac anatomy and physiology, one might think that EKG interpretation had undergone significant refinement since that classic 1958 study. Some thirty years later, however, a second study found that although agreement levels between cardiologists had improved slightly, the far more troublesome measure, doctors' disagreement with themselves, now occurred as much as a quarter of the time.* I read Patrick's EKG the day he came in with chest pain, and I saw no evidence of a

---

*The cardiologists disagreed with their own readings between 10 and 23.2 percent of the time.[4]

heart attack. The following day a cardiologist and an internist read the same EKG—the first agreed with me, the second didn't.

What these studies show is a problem with precision, or reproducibility. Although ideally we would like to measure the accuracy, or correctness, of each physician, this can be an extremely complicated measurement.* But precision, agreement between physicians, is easily measurable. Precision therefore becomes an excellent surrogate marker for accuracy, because in order to be consistently correct, one must first be consistent. To state the obvious, lack of consistency guarantees some inaccuracy. When doctors disagree half the time, then somebody is wrong at least half the time. During Patrick's stay in the hospital he was on the verge of a full-blown heart attack the whole time, and we missed it. Later, when we reviewed Patrick's EKGs, tests, and autopsy results, we still were baffled; we still came to no consensus on the interpretations. With a disease so important, so common, and so difficult to identify, it's disturbing that Patrick's care—and perhaps his survival—were determined by factors on which none of us seem able to agree. And the situation is all too common.

Lily was twenty-three years old, over three hundred pounds, and wincing. Seven days after her gastric bypass operation for obesity, it took six of us to transfer her from the ambulance stretcher to our gurney. After morphine, a normal CAT scan of her abdomen, a chest X-ray that

---

*This is particularly true in the case of heart attacks because of the many features that are computed in the physician's mind that impact a final diagnosis (e.g., examination, EKG, patient history, demographics, community, risk factors, circumstances, experience). Measuring the accuracy of each of these components is complicated and prone to error. In addition, in many cases there isn't necessarily a "correct" answer in reading EKGs, which makes accuracy a judgment call rather than a fact—precisely the problem we're attempting to avoid.

showed only a subtle area of haziness in one lung, and normal blood tests, Lily's abdominal pain persisted.

A consulting surgical resident and I argued about the likely source of her pain.

"It's a week after abdominal surgery and her abdominal pain is her primary complaint. This just seems like postoperative pain," I said. "Or maybe, just maybe, that's a postoperative pneumonia on that X-ray."

The surgical resident held his ground. "I'm just saying it's possible—gastric bypass patients have high pulmonary embolism rates, and she looks short of breath to me."

"If she has a pulmonary embolism," I said, irritated that he wasn't taking responsibility for the problem, "I'll eat my hat."

Lily had a CAT scan of her chest to see if we could determine what was causing the haziness on her X-ray. The scan showed a massive blood clot—a pulmonary embolism—lodged in a blood vessel precisely where the haziness in her X-ray had been.

Inconsistency isn't unique to the diagnosis of heart problems. As common as heart attacks are (about a million per year in the United States), pneumonia, an infection in the tissue of the lung, is five times more common. Diagnosing pneumonia is quite different from diagnosing heart attacks. For one thing, heart attacks are most often diagnosed on the basis of symptoms (what patients tell us they feel) rather than signs (what we find on a physical examination), while in the diagnosis of pneumonia, signs are often more important than symptoms. And in contrast to heart attacks, there's a simple test that generally cinches the diagnosis of pneumonia: the chest X-ray.* Therefore

---

*Some pneumonias are not visible on chest X-rays, but physicians tend to rely on the chest X-ray as the final say in most cases.

the difficult decision is often not which patients have pneumonia, but which patients should have the next step after examination, the chest X-ray. For this, physicians rely heavily on physical examination of the lungs.

One would like to think that the physical examination of patients' lungs, particularly by physicians using stethoscopes, should be fairly consistent. Stethoscopes are, after all, finely crafted precision instruments. Iconic images from Norman Rockwell paintings show the doctor holding his stethoscope (or, famously, listening through the stethoscope to the chest of a young girl's doll). In medical school my classmates and I were given audiotapes of lung sounds, and we watched training videos about using stethoscopes to identify abnormal lung sounds. Later, we were sent out to the wards to listen to every lung we could find. So how much variation can there be in how we interpret lung sounds?

In two separate studies, physicians were asked to examine a patient while paying particular attention to the lung examination—including listening with a stethoscope, tapping the chest, and touching to feel vibrations. This comprehensive pulmonary assessment was repeated on many patients who were being assessed for possible pneumonia. In both studies, physicians consistently disagreed about the presence of signs that might indicate pneumonia.[5]

The results were as troubling as those for heart attacks, and numerically they're worse. They suggest that when the decision to obtain a chest X-ray is based on signs, many patients with pneumonia do not get a chest X-ray, while many without pneumonia do. Perhaps, then, the answer is just to order more chest X-rays when pneumonia is considered. But as in the case of Lily, it's never as simple as it should be. When the surgical resident listened to Lily's lungs, he heard nothing abnormal, but I felt that I did. So we both looked closely at Lily's chest X-ray in order to decide what to do next. Perhaps, at least, the presence of pneumonia on a chest X-ray is something physicians can agree on?

No such luck: experienced doctors will disagree about important X-ray findings, pneumonia included, approximately 20 percent of the time.[6] And the problem is not just the physicians' level of expertise in reading X-rays. Radiologists—physicians who've dedicated their careers to the art of interpreting X-rays—are the true experts, but in an ingenious study of the precision of chest X-ray interpretation performed in the mid-twentieth century, three prominent radiologists were asked to interpret approximately thirty chest X-rays and demonstrated, unsurprisingly, poor agreement. What these doctors didn't know was that every set of thirty X-rays in the study was actually ten X-rays repeated three times over. As with the cardiologists reading EKGs, these radiologists disagreed with themselves almost as often as they disagreed with one another.[7]

Lily's chest X-ray had shown a subtle hint of a problem, and since we couldn't agree, we obtained a CAT scan of her chest, a three-dimensional view of the lungs that can often see pulmonary emboli (blood clots). Lily's blood clot was a large one, and it took high doses of blood-thinning medicine for her to get better, but much to my relief, she did. In Lily's case the primary disagreement had been between two physicians about one patient. But many times the disagreements in medicine can run much deeper, be much more public, and involve much larger groups.

"It's Angela again," Mary, the nurse, said as she handed me the chart. It was my first shift at a small hospital outside Pittsburgh. Mary leaned

in. *"Frequent flyer, big-time. She's here twice a week at least. She'll torture you unless she gets narcotics."*

I found Angela, sixty-five years old and looking thirty years older than that, behind a curtain. The lights were off and she was holding the right side of her head, moaning. "Doctor, mucho, mucho dolor. Mi cabeza." *She rocked back and forth, eyes squeezed shut.*

After examining her, I ordered a migraine medicine to be given through her IV and explained in my broken Spanish that she would feel better soon. Angela waved me away.

Mary looked at me when she saw the order. "She'll spend the whole night here, you know, if you don't just give her Demerol."

"Let's try this first," I said.

Twenty minutes later I felt a hand on my shoulder and saw a smile out of the corner of my eye. "Gracias, muchas gracias, doctor. No dolor. Gracias." *Angela virtually pranced out of the emergency department, with a prescription in her hand.*

Angela is one of at least 30 million Americans who suffer from migraine headaches, many of which lead to emergency department or physician office visits. Watching the extreme suffering that migraines can cause is difficult, but it's also uplifting to see how effective some treatments can be. There is, however, disagreement about which migraine treatments are the most effective.

In 2002 one of the world's leading sources of medical information, *The New England Journal of Medicine,* published an article called "Migraine—Current Understanding and Treatment." The article reviewed research on migraines and recommended the "triptans," a fairly new group of medications, as the best and most effective treatment for acute migraine attacks. In fact, the review dedicated more than half of its eleven pages to an indepth discussion of the triptans, medicines developed by pharmaceutical companies specifically for migraine treatment. But the article was followed by letters from wide-ranging sources questioning the recommendation. It was also met with consternation in the emergency medicine community, where a class of medications called "antiemetics" are most commonly used for migraine treatment. Antiemetics are what worked for Angela, but despite this success, my emergency physician colleagues and I wondered if we'd been doing it wrong all along.

The *NEJM*'s recommendation of the triptans is, it turns out, consistent with the American Academy of Neurology's recommendations[*]—and it was headache experts from the field of neurology who wrote the *NEJM* article. On the other hand, utilizing antiemetics is consistent with the recommendations of the Canadian Headache Society,[8] and also consistent with recent migraine recommendations from experts in the field of emergency medicine.[9] The experts, it appears, disagree. But it turns out that this disagreement is easier to deconstruct than some others. It appears to be partly explained by an odd bit of "parochialism," and partly explained in the fine print of the *NEJM*'s review.

Medical parochialism, in which practices range from place to place and, as in this case, from specialty to specialty, is common. Migraine doctors—neurologists with additional specialized training—and emergency physicians both see and treat migraine patients every day. The difference is that neurologists see patients who have migraines, while emergency physicians see patients who are having migraines. The training and experience of a migraine specialist tends to be most concentrated on the preven-

---

[*]Note that one of the authors of the *NEJM* review is one of the authors of the AAN's migraine guidelines and that these guidelines were funded by triptan pharmaceutical companies. This guideline is available as a download at www.aan.com. Accessed 2/08.

tion and treatment of *future* migraines, while the training and experience of an emergency physician is concentrated on the treatment of acute migraines as they are occurring.

Acute migraine studies have, therefore, commonly been done by emergency physicians in emergency departments, and some twenty-five years ago one of these studies led to a fortuitous discovery. Because migraines are frequently associated with nausea and vomiting, giving migraine medicines in the form of a pill was not always possible. Researchers, therefore, tried giving patients with acute migraines a dose of "antiemetic" (that is, antivomiting) medication before giving the migraine medicine. Much to the surprise of the researchers, the migraines often quickly dissipated soon after the antiemetics—but before the study pills had been given. In follow-up studies, dozens of which were published in emergency medicine journals, virtually all of the antiemetic medicines were found to be highly effective for halting acute migraine attacks. The antiemetics have since become a widespread first choice for migraine treatment in emergency departments around the world.

Neurologists, on the other hand, are frequently unaware of these studies. Many physicians read primarily the medical literature that focuses on their specialty and is relevant to their patients. Emergency medicine doctors, for instance, know comparatively little about studies of medications helpful in the long-term care of migraine patients. The *NEJM* review article, however, written by three neurologists, attempts to address both the long-term care of migraine patients (mostly a neurology domain) and the care of acute attacks (mostly an emergency medicine domain). While the review seems to nicely summarize research on the prevention of migraines, it unfortunately fails to note a single study about how and where physicians treat acute migraines most—in an emergency department.

This lapse, a likely product of medical parochialism, would be unimportant if the triptans and the antiemetics were very similar in their effects, and indeed they have similar success rates for stopping migraines. The triptans, however, have serious side-effect problems, including more "rebound" headaches (on the day after treatment) and blood-vessel side effects that make them inappropriate for anyone with possible heart disease. But the biggest and most universal difference is cost. The triptans are a new class of designer medications, many of which are still on patent and therefore unavailable in a generic form, and so they cost up to one hundred times more than the antiemetics. Despite antiemetics' clear economic and health benefits, the *NEJM*'s theoretically comprehensive review of acute migraine treatment mentions them once. Almost unbelievably, the sole mention of antiemetics is a suggestion that they might be useful in the role to which they had been relegated decades earlier, before they had been studied for use in migraines—as a medicine to treat nausea so that the patient is able to ingest the triptan.

A difference in knowledge and experience between neurology and emergency medicine helps to explain this disagreement, but one must wonder if there are other factors in play. After all, the three authors of the *NEJM* article are world-renowned, highly published experts on migraine. Could they have fallen so deeply into the trap of single-specialty knowledge? Could they be unaware of the antiemetics, unaware of the Canadian Headache Society recommendations? I contacted one of the authors of the migraine review article and asked about the recommendations. He defended his review as scientifically well founded and said that it wasn't "about treatment in the ED." Nothing in the article (which claims to be a comprehensive review of migraine treatment for medical providers) reflects this limitation, however, and the antiemetics have been proven as effective as the triptans in every setting in which they've been studied, not just ED.

I also told him that I wondered if there were more to the omission of the antiemetics than parochialism. In the "disclosures" section at the end of the article, in fine print, the three authors report having received money in the form of grants and consulting fees from pharmaceutical corporations—each of the seven pharmaceutical companies that manufacture the seven triptan medications mentioned by name in the review. Critics of pharmaceutical company funding for medical research have often claimed that it leads to biased results, and indeed studies have shown that industry-funded reports yield results favorable to the funding companies much more often than non-industry reports.[10] While this may not be evidence that the funding they received affected their recommendations, the appearance of a conflict is certainly present.*

The pharmaceutical corporations marketing the triptans have developed an effective set of strategies to overcome the fact that there are cheaper, safer, more effective alternatives for migraine treatment. One strategy has been the enrollment of huge numbers of patients in massive triptan studies. Despite the fact that these triptan studies are of no higher quality than antiemetic studies, and have demonstrated no better efficacy for triptans than for antiemetics, the studies seem very impressive, because they contain a hundred thousand patients (the antiemetic trials

---

*The study author's responses to me make clear that he does not believe that funding influenced his review. As noted earlier, studies have shown that bias often results from subconscious processes that are not identifiable to those experiencing them. Therefore, there is nothing here to suggest intentionally misleading conclusions; there is simply evidence of a strong impetus for (perhaps subconscious) bias—in this case research funding and other support.

include only a few thousand patients). A second marketing strategy has been the enlistment of experts in the field of headache medicine. Research grants, "consulting" fees, and highly paid engagements to speak publicly (often about the triptans) have all been given to respected experts in the field. Headache experts, leaders in their narrow field, often teach in major academic centers and publish research, and therefore have considerable influence. They are also occasionally asked to write reviews for the *NEJM*.

Another clever strategy used to promote the use of triptans has been the careful avoidance of head-to-head comparisons between the triptans and the antiemetics. Until recently, despite enrolling gargantuan numbers of migraine patients in hundreds of trials comparing triptans to placebos, only nine trials had rigorously compared triptans to any other medicines, and none of these directly compared triptans and antiemetics.* In 2004, however, two of the authors of the 2002 *NEJM* article published a review of these nine trials. They reported what the data showed: that the triptans were no better than any other migraine medications (including some cheap over-the-counter remedies). But in a remarkably brash example of circular logic, the authors then laid out a detailed argument for why the data must be flawed, since it's well known that the triptans are better.[11]

In an effort to address the question more directly, a research group that included one of the authors of the *NEJM*, sponsored by the National Institutes of Health compared the best-known

---

*It is difficult to determine precisely how the medical community or the FDA came to see the triptans as an effective or essential medication for migraines based on studies comparing them to placebos. In order to prove its worth, a new medication should be compared to the existing standard care for a condition, not placebos. Therefore the issue of whether or not the triptans are better than other medicines used for migraine was largely sidestepped except in this small group of nine studies.

triptan medicine to a common antiemetic medicine for patients having acute migraines. In every measurable way, the antiemetic was equal or superior to the triptan. Moreover, it cost $4 per dose, compared to $60 per dose for the triptan.[12]

One unanswered question about this medical disagreement is how and why an influential medical journal allowed the publication of a migraine review that is, at best, incomplete and unproven. Another is whether or not the authors of the review intentionally ignored data. Perhaps not. Perhaps they are simply researchers rather than clinicians. Some physicians are experienced acute migraine doctors, seeing patients with migraine attacks every day. And some physicians, occasionally those who are highly published and known for their expertise, rarely see patients. In addition, as noted above, neurologists more often meet patients like Angela after her doctor has referred them, or after they have had multiple emergency department visits. They see only difficult, refractory cases, and they generally see patients at a time when they're having no pain. Therefore they may never see Angela when she's holding her head and pleading for quiet and darkness. This discrepancy may also explain the puzzling decision of the American Academy of Neurology to recommend the triptans first for acute attacks.*

Perhaps and perhaps. But the question of whether that research money has affected an influential scientific publication in this case is hard to avoid, and as a source of medical disagreement it may become common.

• • •

---

*Last chapter's discussion of professional medical society guidelines is certainly applicable here as well. As an additional note, one of the authors of the AAN guidelines was an author of the *NEJM* migraine review, and the development of the guidelines was done with "funding and support" from five different pharmaceutical corporations that make triptan drugs (see p. 33 of the guideline).

At least the influence of marketing and medical colloquialism are tangible reasons for discord, and they're theoretically fixable. In the case of signs and symptoms of diseases like heart attack and pneumonia, however, disagreement among physicians means that the science of physical examination is disappointingly unscientific. Physical diagnosis is yet another area of modern medicine in which the breadth of our knowledge is frighteningly small in comparison to the vast sea of truth that has yet to be charted. In the case of EKGs and chest X-rays, it stands to reason that if experts are unable to consistently agree on the results of a test, then either the test is flawed or the expertise is flawed. In either case the result is uncertainty. And while it may seem as if the problem is the physician, very often it is not. It is, simply put, asking too much for us humans to be perfectly consistent in the way we report our pain, or the way we understand the symptoms of others, or the way we read a test's results. We are inconsistent creatures. As Aldous Huxley once said, "Consistency is contrary to nature, contrary to life. The only completely consistent people are dead."

What, then, is the solution? Where the reaches of our science have yet to satisfy the needs of our patients, where gray areas and disagreements dominate, we have often sought second opinions. This course of action has merit. But as we've seen, experts often disagree, and the opinions of two disagreeing experts may not always bring us closer to an accurate answer. A potentially more honest approach is not out of our reach: we can show our cards. Disagreements can become open points of discussion rather than hidden points of controversy debated quietly among physicians. The uncertainty suggested by the presence of disagreement or controversy can be acknowledged. In most cases, where there is no clear right answer, the values of the patient—the one ostensibly being benefited—should be driving decisions.

The greatest barrier to this approach is also the most obvious, and that is our instinct to hide uncertainty and to ignore or minimize disagreement. In the case of Luke's plantar fasciitis, the best treatments are yet unknown. In making our suggestions, both Luke's physician and I were improvising, relying on traditional and common—but unproven—techniques. But Luke didn't know that, and he and others haven't traditionally been told that many of the everyday questions in medicine are answered this way.

We've been unaccountably quiet on this issue, and patients have been led to believe that when a physician listens to their heart, the cold metal that they feel is the price for hard science, a moment of clear and unencumbered physiologic insight. The dishonesty of this myth is perpetuated in the iconic images of the doctor listening to a patient's heart through the mighty stethoscope, or examining an X-ray and confidently pronouncing a diagnosis. The tender acts of medicine that Norman Rockwell portrayed were no more scientific than the motions and colors of the brush that painted them. Hippocrates referred to medicine as "the Art," a reality that we often shun or attempt to hide, rather than acknowledge and accept. We have no reason to hide the Art. For while complete agreement is rarely possible, complete honesty almost always is.

4

WE DON'T TALK

I was jarred from sleep by a high-pitched tweeting sound, followed by a woman's raspy upstate–New York accent: "Need a crew for a call, full crew for a call . . . One-twenty-three Hudson Street, Johnson City . . . Seventy-one-year-old male, not breathing . . . Full crew for a call."

The clock read 6:35 A.M. I had arrived home twenty minutes earlier from the ambulance station where I worked as a professional paramedic. Now the volunteer squad in town was paging for a call just a few blocks away. I sat up and shook my head like a wet dog, threw on jeans and a T-shirt, and grabbed my portable radio.

"One-fifteen-Edward to central, responding from Harrison Street."

"Thank you, one-fifteen-Edward." Though we knew each other only through the filter of radio communications, I always felt like there was palpable relief in Nancy's voice when I responded to the calls that no one else did. "Fire is en route as well."

"Ten-four." I frowned. The local fire department was famously untrained for medical emergencies, so I wondered why they would have any interest in this. On the other hand, they were very, very enthusiastic.

Not realizing how close I was, I got in the car, drove around the corner, saw the address, and got out of the car. A rusty blue Ford Bronco with a flashing red-light bar on top pulled up at the same time I did, sirens winding down. A small, stout man emerged from the vehicle running at top speed. He grabbed a green bag from the back of his truck without so much as a moment's deceleration.

"Hi, Chief, how're you?" I spoke slowly, in the false hope that my calm would influence the fire chief.

He barked, "Let's hit it!" as he ran up the front steps. He swung open the door and ran inside. I hoped it was the right house.

I followed him, tentatively, into a modest living room where a middle-aged husband and wife, two teenaged boys, and an elderly woman all stood. The woman pointed. "He's in the back. Hurry, please." Indeed the chief accelerated from top speed, and I tried to keep up as he raced into a back bedroom.

An elderly man in pajamas was lying on the bed with his back to us, not moving. Chief opened his bag as I touched the man's shoulder. When there was no response, I tried to roll him onto his back. He didn't roll easily. And when he did, everything rolled at once.

Chief looked up. "What the . . . ?"

The man had rigor mortis, which meant he had probably died hours earlier, in his sleep. He rolled like a Madame Tussauds rendering, and settled back into position on the bed when I let go.

"Yeah, Chief, looks like we're late for this one." I took a deep breath, steeling myself to tell the family.

"Wait a sec, he's dead?" Chief asked me loudly.

I gestured at him to keep it down. "Yeah, Chief, he's gone."

Chief tried to roll the man himself. He yelled, "Aw jeez, he is dead."

"Um, yeah . . ." He walked past me out of the room. "Chief? Where are you . . . ?"

The older woman held her hands over her mouth and asked about her husband. "Is he all right? Will he be okay?"

I came out of the room just behind the chief, a step late. "Okay?" said the chief. "He's dead. I mean, he is dead, really dead. Jeez he's dead."

"Chief," I pleaded, "could I . . . ?" The chief looked at me, then turned back to the woman, whose eyes were growing wider.

"Heeeeeee's dead dead. I mean, what did you . . . he's been . . . he's just plain dead. Wow, he's dead." I slipped past them and out into the street while the chief continued elaborating in the same vein.

I held the radio to my mouth discreetly as I got in the car. "One-fifteen-Edward to Communications. Fire's reporting code black; cancel all incoming units."

"Ten-four," Nancy chirped. "I never heard you call 'on scene.' Did you make it?"

I paused to think about that one. "Negative, negative, Communications. Chief's on scene, he's got this one."

"Ten-four, one-fifteen-Edward. Thanks again. And get some sleep."

"Roger, I'll try."

Thus ended my first outstanding lesson in how not to deliver bad news. The exuberant fire chief's approach had made me cringe, and it didn't take a genius to see that there must be a bet-

ter way to break bad news. Over the years I've had many oppor-
tunities to practice, read about, and consider my own approach
to family and patient notification of diagnoses, deaths, and
injuries. But beyond raw experience, beyond throwing physicians into the fire to blunder along haplessly until they're finally
(one hopes) facile at this skill, how do we teach doctors the art
of delivering bad news? The easy answer is, we don't.

The lack of instruction in such a crucial area is perplexing
when one considers that communication between people is the
foundation of medicine, and it was the primary method by
which the highly successful Hippocrates plied the Art in ancient
Greece. Empathy, socialization, and cultural sensitivity are all
desirable physician traits, all are critical for success in the healing
arts, and all depend on the ability to communicate. And yet a
comprehensive review of patients' opinions of primary care
physicians between 1996 and 2000 found that patients increasingly sense deterioration in physicians' communication skills, as
well as their "interpersonal treatment" and their ability to gain
patient trust.[1] Poor communication is a major contributor to the
increasing distance between doctors and patients.

Not a dinner party passes without someone telling me an
atrocious tale about an oblivious physician who insulted, ignored,
demeaned, dismissed, or otherwise mistreated them. One is
prone to wonder whether the doctors in these anecdotes were
even human, and the root issue is virtually always communication. While such stories may occasionally be colored by personal
biases or perhaps one-sided perspectives, it's too often true that
basic social skills seem to have been lost somewhere along the
path of medical education, and there are a number of places on
this path where this may have occurred. During medical school
and residency a physician's time for psychological health, family,
and social outlets dwindles to near nothing. Recent studies of

medical students have demonstrated an alarmingly high rate of depression and mental health problems, and residency training after medical school is typically even more consuming.[2]

The potential for personal discontent combined with a lack of training in communication skills like delivering bad news translates into poor people skills. As residents, my classmates and I were shown a videotape of a mock patient scenario that included the notification of a family about an individual's death. The video was about twenty minutes long, and though it was cinematically crude, it was carefully made and it elegantly described the important principles of family notification. I'm now in a position where I frequently deliver news about illness, injury, or death—and yet those twenty minutes were the beginning and the end of my formal training in family notification.

How important is the sensitive communication of bad news? Very important. The quality of doctor-patient communication appears to be a prime factor in both short- and long-term psychological adjustment for patients and families—even when the news is terrible.* Numerous studies attest to patients' desires to feel empathy and concern from their physician, but in moments of crisis doctors are often perceived to be cold or unemotional. Perhaps it's the image of the scientist that we're attempting to uphold, or maybe it is our normal and appropriate coping mechanism, our attempt to distance ourselves from the daily tragedies to which some of us are exposed. Regardless of the reason, the

---

*Interestingly, there is another attribute to poor communication of bad news: good patient communication skills also appear to be important for the psychological well-being of the *physician*. In a British study published in 1995, it was found that significantly higher levels of job dissatisfaction, distress, and factors related to occupational burnout were more likely in those who had been insufficiently trained in communication skills.[3]

truth is that doctors feel a great deal in these situations and such moments take a toll on us. In fact, our feelings about the quality of such interactions are tied closely to our sense of success or failure. One study of oncologists showed that when a physician thinks he's communicated poorly, he tends to feel that he's failed medically as well.[4]

Moreover, physicians' assessments of their communication success or failure may have an impact on their choices of treatment. In the study noted above, a sense of having failed a patient was statistically associated with the use of chemotherapy for that patient—even when the patient was already in the final phase of a terminal illness. This is an unnecessary (and potentially damaging and uncomfortable) measure, and likely reflects a physician's feelings of desperation or inadequacy. In popular media, we've all seen portrayals of vigorous and emotional CPR being performed by a physician who refuses to "allow" a patient to die. While this is almost always unrealistic, conceptually it is not far removed from a futile, last-ditch round of chemotherapy in an already terminal cancer patient. Doctors who haven't communicated well with dying patients are more likely to make poor, even desperate decisions about medical care.

Most doctors aren't oncologists, and infrequently find themselves informing a family or patient of tragic news. Therefore most effects of poor communication are much more subtle than mishandled family notification or unnecessary chemotherapy. More often, the impact of poor communication is insidious. Even a problem as simple as a twisted ankle can create doctor-patient problems that have systemwide repercussions.

It was nearing the end of a seemingly endless shift during residency, and I rubbed my eyes as I picked up the chart. Alane, a young woman with an ankle injury, was waiting in Room 2 to be seen by a physician, and she had arrived by ambulance. I took a deep breath and shook my head. An ambulance for an ankle injury?

When I entered the room I took note of how pleasantly comfortable Alane appeared, and I looked back at the chart to note that she had told the nurse that her pain was a "nine out of ten"—nearly the worst pain she could ever imagine. I shook my head again. "How can we help you, ma'am?" I offered.

"Well, I took a turn with my ankle going from the third to the bottom step, and now . . ."

She pointed to her right ankle, which looked fine to me, if perhaps slightly swollen. I nodded, and pressed haphazardly and disinterestedly on a few of the bones that make up the ankle joint. She jumped a bit as I touched them, but appeared to have good nerve and blood-vessel function. "Well, I really doubt it's broken. Seems like it's a regular old sprain. I'm not really sure we need X-rays," I said, and then shrugged in resignation. "But I suppose we'll get some just to be sure."

She seemed surprised. "Sprained? Wow. That's a pretty bad sprain, I guess."

"Uh-huh. Well, we can get you some pain medicine if you want, and I'll come back after the X-rays are done." I set her chart aside and forgot to order the pain medicine.

Later, after I found her X-rays on the viewing machine, I stared at them for five minutes, checking and rechecking to see if somehow Alane's name had gotten on the wrong X-ray. The ankle bones in the X-rays were dislocated, and "comminuted"—shattered.

I entered the room sheepishly, holding the X-rays, and told Alane. She looked at me quietly and nodded. I spent the next hour giving her strong pain medications, splinting and fixing the dislocation, and then arranging for the surgery that she would need for an ankle so badly broken.

I was tired when I saw Alane, and my judgment was poor. Clouded by her stoicism, my fatigue, and my cynicism about a complaint we see many times every day, I not only lacked empathy, I was dismissive. And I regretted it—not just because she was seriously injured, but because it made my inexperience and bad doctoring abundantly clear. Even if she had turned out to have just a minor ankle sprain, I would've been wrong, and we both knew it.

My communication with Alane was hopelessly unprofessional, and the choice I nearly made—not to get an X-ray—would've been an exceptionally bad one. But in fact such a decision shouldn't even have been possible. Physicians have a highly efficient tool at their disposal for determining who does, and doesn't, need X-rays for ankle injuries. I'm talking about the "Ottawa Ankle Rule" (named for the Canadian capital, where it was developed), a decision rule consisting of five steps. The first four involve the palpation, or pressing, of four well-defined areas on the ankle and foot: the backs of both ankle bones (tibia and fibula), the navicular bone (roughly the dead center of the top of the foot), and the base of the fifth metatarsal bone (the bony prominence where the outside portion of the foot sticks out the farthest). Pressing on these areas should not cause pain if there is no fracture. The fifth step is a single question: Was the patient able to limp on the affected leg right after the injury occurred, and can he limp on it at the time of examination? With these five components, a physician can correctly identify approximately 98–99 percent of ankle fractures, and the 1 percent that may be missed are likely to be unimportant, requiring no treatment.[5] If there's no tenderness at the four areas and a patient can limp after the injury and during examination, for all intents and purposes there's no broken ankle. If I had followed this simple rule, I wouldn't have wondered whether Alane needed an X-ray.

The development of the Ottawa Ankle Rule in 1993 wasn't minor; it was revolutionary. The ten-second evaluation consistently and safely obviates the need for approximately one-quarter of all potential X-rays in a group of patients that requires millions of X-rays per year. But after the Ottawa Ankle Rule was created, and well after it was proven to be extremely effective, researchers found that there was an unexpected and somewhat baffling factor hindering its implementation—most physicians won't use it.[6]

Why not? The answer is complicated, but appears to be based largely in what physicians perceive to be patients' desires: patients often want X-rays, and doctors tend to do what patients want. Studies show that satisfaction with care depends in part upon expectations for care, and physicians feel that patients with ankle injuries often come with the explicit expectation of having an X-ray.

What's a physician to do when a patient wants an X-ray even after the Ottawa Ankle Rule has determined it to be unnecessary? The answer seems self-evident: talk to the patient. If a doctor explains the Ottawa Ankle Rule, describes the costs of X-rays in both time and money, and makes clear the virtually perfect performance of the rule, the problem should be solved. After all, with rare exceptions there's little to be gained from an X-ray if there's no broken bone, since X-rays don't allow one to see injured ligaments, tendons, or other soft tissues. Moreover, studies have demonstrated that satisfaction with treatment for an ankle injury isn't actually related to whether or not an X-ray is taken;[7] satisfaction is related to empathy, concern, and communication. It is widely known, for instance, that if a physician sits in a chair to talk to a patient rather than standing throughout the encounter—even if the length of time with the patient is identical—patients more often feel that the physician was concerned, empathetic, and spent time with them.

But even with the widespread diffusion of the Ottawa Ankle Rule, physicians are still ordering the same number of X-rays, which raises a number of issues. The choice to order an X-ray is almost certainly related to time pressures, since time spent on a conversation describing and explaining the utility of X-rays is physician time, while time spent when a patient is sent to the X-ray area (first to wait and then eventually to be X-rayed by a radiology technician) is patient, technician, and machine time. This choice disregards, of course, the burden of total time and money spent in the system, as well as the bottleneck effect on other patients and physicians when X-rays are ordered. But ultimately it's an individual physician's choice, a method to extract a few precious minutes from a day bursting at its seams.

The choice to order X-rays also reflects, on the part of both physicians and patients, a common overreliance and faith in imaging and blood tests—a deferral to technology. But the deferral is ironic: the 99 percent certainty afforded by the Ottawa Ankle Rule can't even be approached by the comparatively subjective and variable accuracy associated with reading an X-ray.

The fact that physicians commonly order X-rays that they privately acknowledge are medically unnecessary also makes one wonder how often this lack of communication occurs in other areas of medicine. In an attempt to address this question, a research group in California performed a clever study. Over a period of a few months, they sent an actor playing the role of a patient into the offices of thirty-nine different physicians. The actor told each physician that she was suffering from fatigue (but no other symptoms) and explained that her close friend had multiple sclerosis, which had made her concerned that she herself might have multiple sclerosis. The actor then specifically requested a brain MRI, an expensive and unnecessary test. (The ordering of an MRI in this situation would be inappropriate for many reasons, the simplest being that isolated and generalized fatigue is virtually never MS.) If the physician then refused to arrange for an MRI, the actor-patient requested referral to a neurologist, another expensive and unnecessary step.

How did the physicians respond? In nearly a third of the encounters the physician agreed to order an MRI or to potentially do so at a later visit. Of the physicians who stood fast on the MRI, over half then compromised by referring the patient to a neurologist. The great majority of doctors therefore ultimately capitulated to a patient's uneducated requests for expensive and unnecessary medical tests or referrals, rather than invest time in communicating.

Clearly the fictitious patient was anxious about having MS, but since it's not contagious (she couldn't have contracted it from a friend) and virtually never manifests as isolated fatigue, reassurance should have been simple. The designers of the study tracked how often the doctors attempted to offer this reassurance. Generally, of course, they didn't. When they did, the actor (as part of the script) was then easily reassured, and both the imaging tests and the referral became unnecessary. But most of the physicians never got to this part of the script.

An additional note on the actor-patient study: four of the physicians (roughly 10 percent) chose their own approach to her concerns about MS and her request for an MRI. One told the patient she was being irrational, a second called her "paranoid," a third told her that she had a "psychic imbalance," and a fourth ignored her request entirely.[8]

Time pressures, faith in technology, system inefficiency, poor communication, and patient demands (sometimes from inflexible or poorly informed patients) all contribute to the study's results. And each of these root problems seems likely to worsen rather than improve. Lack of communication begets lack of communication, a downward spiral closely tied to medicine's movement away from contact and toward technology, a movement embraced by patients and doctors alike. Both groups crave the safety and the seemingly unimpeachable science represented by blood tests, X-rays, and pills.

Besides the obvious labor and financial burdens that result from being hypnotized by the monuments of science, there's an additional and much greater cost—the displacement of the Art of doctoring. In the field of medical education, this lost Art has been noted and discussed for nearly the past hundred years. Policy makers and leaders in medical education describe the prototype physician model as being "curious," "compassionate," and "moral," and yet none of these attributes appears to be seriously attended to in medical education—and they never have been.[9] How can a physician understand how to genuinely communicate or empathize with others when he can barely understand himself?

Our class sat in the lecture hall, uncommonly attentive. Playing on the screen in front of us was a video of a woman undergoing a detailed breast and pelvic examination. Oddly, the woman looked into the camera and narrated as she was examined. She was a "professional patient," and in addition to being regularly poked and prodded by hapless medical students at our institution, she played the lead role in this educational videotape. It was indeed educational. And strange.

After the video had finished, we stood in the hallway outside the lecture hall. There was scattered nervous laughter and some awkward discussion, with many of the female students expressing amazement—"How does she do that?"—or just shaking their heads.

The male students fell into two distinct groups—one silent, the other not so. Our class had a number of what we referred to as "six-year wonders," students who participated in a combined college/medical school program that included only two years of undergraduate study, followed immediately by enrollment in medical school. Many of them had begun their medical education at the age of nineteen or twenty, and it was one of these students (male) who blurted out, with a sour grimace, "That didn't turn me on at all!"

The hallway fell silent, and one of the oldest female students in the class fixed him with a powerful stare. After a few seconds of burning a hole through him, she walked over and said, her voice thick with disgust, "But you see, boy genius, it's not supposed to. Get it?"

He got it. We all got it.

What does a confused medical student have to do with a doctor's inability to communicate? Both are part of the same tattered educational foundation. In order for one to be comfortable communicating, one must first be comfortable. The basic comfort and confidence that come from understanding professional context and professional communication isn't something that's generally taught in the House of Medicine. As a result, one of our deepest secrets is that physicians are often uncomfortable.

My class's awkward hallway moment was testament to this discomfort. While some take to professional roles naturally and easily, many do not. During my medical education nobody told us how to professionally interpret and reintegrate the social standards that we had lived with all our lives. No one spoke to our class about the sociosexual implications of the film, and no one introduced it with a parental talk. No one explained what we might feel or see, and—perhaps most important—no one told us how a physician learns to set aside a lifetime of human interaction and socialization in the blink of an eye in order to become a professional. No one ever told us how we might transform our social, human selves into our doctor selves.

The transition is complicated and difficult, and it requires specific attention and skill. When I was in medical school, no one taught me how to keep from gawking openly in front of a patient with a visually striking wound, or how to remain quiet and politely attentive while a patient with a severe stutter speaks, or how to deal with physical attraction (in either direction) during interaction with patients. This can be difficult to explain, particularly to laypeople, who understandably prefer to see physicians as persons capable of suspending human tendencies like anger, fear, and physical attraction. One analogy I have used in teaching students is that of the bank teller. The first few hours, or even days, of handling great quantities of cash may seem personally challenging for the teller, a test of his restraint. He may desire or covet the money, or be tempted to devise clandestine methods to horde it for himself. But soon enough (and perhaps from the very beginning for some), professional instincts and routines make such restraint unnecessary. Handling money becomes a part of everyday existence. While money may be something bank tellers desire, it is soon ingrained in a teller's mind that *this* money is quite distinct from what they desire.

This explanation works for some and not for others, and for some who have excellent professional instincts it's unnecessary. But the issues are difficult, and the complicating factors of taboos, preconceptions, and everyday social repression often compound the difficulty. While learning how to work with and around these issues requires the most directed teaching, medical education instead tends to skip over them entirely.

A "perspective" piece for *The New England Journal of Medicine* in 2005 pointed out a telling void in the current practice of medicine: there's no uniform professional standard for the many "how-to's" of patient modesty and discretion in the physical examination of patients.[10] For instance, should there be same-sex chaperones present for examinations of potentially private body areas? And which areas—the waistline, the groin, the buttock? No standard has been set in medical practice that answers this question. There's no policy, no approved or disseminated guideline, no ethical writ, and no accepted convention. Thus it should be no surprise that no cohesive message is imparted to medical students. As with most nebulous and deficient areas in our field, medical education is only as confused as medical practice.

Social and cultural confusion is awkward and difficult, but it can also be dangerous. Beyond decisions about exposing someone's waistline during a medical examination lie broader challenges to doctor-patient communication, and as our country becomes more culturally diverse, this problem will only increase. Where communication is limited, good medicine—sometimes lifesaving medicine—is also limited.

Kim, a Chinese woman of thirty-six, was standing in an elevator when she doubled over with sudden and severe abdominal pain. Her husband called an ambulance immediately, and watched helplessly as she lost consciousness. Paramedics found her semiconscious, with a blood pressure of 60/20 and a diffusely tender abdomen.

On arrival in our emergency department, she had a low blood pressure, her heart was racing, and though more lucid, she remained groggy.

Her husband told us she had undergone in vitro fertilization ten weeks earlier, a procedure that we immediately recognized put her at high risk for an ectopic pregnancy, the accidental implantation of a fertilized egg somewhere other than in the uterus. This errant implantation often happens inside one of the fallopian tubes, and unless identified early, such a pregnancy will eventually rupture the tube, causing bleeding and requiring an emergency operation. Patients who don't have this operation early can die quickly from hemorrhage.

In order to determine if there was internal bleeding, we performed an emergency ultrasound on Kim, which showed blood gathering in her abdominal cavity. A rapid blood test also confirmed that her blood counts were low. Indeed, she had all the classic signs and symptoms of a ruptured ectopic pregnancy.

Despite the severity of her condition, Kim was stoic, fitting a cultural profile that is well known in medicine. It's widely asserted that while individuals from some cultures are often highly expressive of suffering or discomfort, Chinese individuals tend to be less so than others. Kim looked uncomfortable but didn't complain of pain, though she admitted to it when asked. She didn't request anything except her husband's presence, and he was openly thankful for our care as he sat at her side holding her hand.

When the gynecology team examined Kim minutes after her arrival, her blood pressure was back to normal because of the intravenous fluids we had given her. Due to this normal blood pressure, they decided to wait for the results of further tests before determining a course of action. The emergency medicine residents and I recommended immediate surgery, and I spoke at length with the gynecologist in charge, pointing out the evidence of ongoing internal bleeding, but to no avail. It was perhaps "just a cyst," the gynecologist felt, not a ruptured ectopic pregnancy. The decision was firm—to await further tests.

When a third consecutive test confirmed worsening internal bleed-

ing and shock, Kim was taken to the operating room, where a ruptured fallopian tube due to an ectopic pregnancy was confirmed—more than twelve hours after she arrived.

Fortunately, other than a longer stay in the hospital and more blood transfusions, Kim suffered only minor ill effects from her twelve-hour delay, and she walked out of the hospital in less than a week. She was lucky to be alive. But why did such a long delay occur? Looking back, even the gynecologists were baffled. As one of them pointed out, if a written examination for gynecology competence had described a fictional patient like Kim, even a medical student would know to instantly rush her to the operating room. When I asked a number of the gynecologists, trainees, and attending physicians what the determining factor was in delaying her operation, there was a recurring comment: *"She didn't seem to have much pain."*

In medical school we read articles, books, and short stories about varying cultural and individual responses to illness, and then we participated in group discussions. We talked about the cultural "sick role" and the common variations in the expression and understanding of pain. We dissected the cultural inculcations that explain why some individuals arrive three days into their illness while others arrive in the first few minutes, and we noted how people of Asian cultures typically express pain when compared to others. We discussed such issues until it seemed we were blue in the face, and I recall some students eventually becoming fed up with the topic. But the journey from medical school to attending physician is a long one, and I don't recall a moment of residency training spent on what medical education experts now call "cultural competence."

For a telling demonstration one needs only to search the biomedical literature for studies focusing on cultural understanding in medical education. Few can be found. An editorial in *The New England Journal of Medicine* in 2004 discussed the importance of cultural competence in medical education but was unable to cite a single study, and concluded that "cultural competence is still at an early stage."[11] A year later the journal published a second editorial emphasizing the importance of the topic but scolding those who currently teach cultural competence in medicine for not first recognizing the powerful and pervasive culture of biomedical science that affects their own perceptions and approaches. The author called the current teachings "old wine in new bottles," and described cultural understanding as "one of the most persistent problems in medical education."[12]

Poor communication is making everyone unhappy. Professional discontent among physicians is higher than ever, and patient satisfaction is dropping in tandem.[13] The medical malpractice crisis exemplifies the issue: lawsuits are filed almost exclusively by those who are dissatisfied, and what satisfies people most is communication. Even in the setting of poor outcomes like death and disability, the quality of communication remains the most powerful predictor of lawsuits. When medical errors occur, full disclosure to patients and families—including abandonment of all secrecy and prompt acceptance of blame—is the most effective known strategy for reducing lawsuits. Fewer claims are filed and smaller awards result.[14] Malpractice claims, therefore, occur because of poor communication, and a culture of malpractice strains communication. Medical malpractice is microcosmic of our larger system's problems and its potential solutions: poor communication is the problem, and good communication is both the prevention and the cure.

• • •

Hippocrates was a communicator. With patients he listened more than he spoke, absorbing and recording exhaustively to understand their desires, their intentions, and their milieu. The state of science and technical know-how in his era made communication his most valuable tool. In our system, communication has been cast aside as a trivial component of medical care and a nonentity in medical education, dwarfed by what we perceive to be the great potency and authority of medical science. While its absence is glaringly obvious to most patients, it remains, paradoxically, largely unspoken among doctors: we don't value communication, we don't appreciate its healing potential, and we don't seriously teach or encourage it.

5

WE PREFER TESTS

*I*t was with some trepidation that I started my first hospital rotation, knowing that my adviser was to be Jon. Jon, a senior student,
was a year ahead of me, a few years older than the average student, and he was a Type 3.

In the first two years of medical school, the classroom years, there
are three species of student. The first sit in the front rows of the lecture
hall. They take detailed notes and ask pointed questions. They are visibly driven. With rare exceptions they spend their afternoons and
evenings in the library.

The second species is slightly more relaxed, sitting farther back in *the classroom among small gaggles of friends. They absorb and share both the academic and social experience of learning, and their afternoons are spent reading in groups, often on grassy fields or in living rooms. The first and second types know each other well. On special occasions they even intermingle. While they may lack a perfect mutual understanding, they respect each other.*

The third type, however, are markedly different from the first two, and much less common. They take medical school as a correspondence course. They're poorly understood, and rarely seen. They (reportedly) read the core material on their own. They appear only when attendance is mandatory, for instance in small group sessions. Even then they're seen fleetingly, only long enough, perhaps, to sign an attendance record.

Because Type 3 students are a perennial topic of conversation, I had heard of Jon. His job as my adviser would be, ostensibly, to ease my transition from the classroom to the hospital. I hoped he at least knew something about the latter.

During the first week I did as my med student handbooks told me: I woke up at 4 A.M. and raced around the hospital, briefly seeing each of my assigned patients before rounds. I checked vital signs, wrote notes in charts, and memorized the morning blood test results in order to give my team a progress report during morning rounds. I spent many hours with my hands behind my back, wearing the short white coat, waiting for the attending physician to begin leading us through the hospital on rounds. The afternoons were spent checking late-arriving lab test results, looking at X-rays and CAT scans, and transcribing the results of all of these tests into the medical chart. Evenings were for reading about my patients' illnesses. During this period and the subsequent weeks, Jon rarely spoke, though he had competent answers to any questions. He appeared amused but always nodded supportively when I recited my crisp patient reports for the team on rounds.

By the end of the first few weeks I had mastered the routine, but I knew that there was something else I should be doing—I just didn't know what it was. The team seemed pleased with my morning summaries, and no one had scolded me. In fact, my interim evaluations were shining. But I had spent minimal time with my patients. I had learned very little about examining or speaking to patients, or diagnosing and treating illness at the bedside. I waited for someone to tell me what I was missing.

In the fourth week, after rounds were over on a particularly long morning, I stood contemplating this missing link. I was beginning to feel frustrated, and it must have been visible. Jon leaned toward me and in a gentle voice, he said, "This is your next two years, man. Settle in."

I had been waiting for this. "What's my next two years? What do you mean?" I asked.

"I mean this." He nodded at the group.

I looked around me and saw an attending physician, a fellow, three resident doctors, two interns, and three medical students, all doing roughly the same thing I was: They rocked back and forth on their heels, or scribbled things into a notepad, or wrote in charts, or punched keys on a computer. They spoke to one another and looked about. Jon, who would later become a well-known family practitioner with an overflowing practice of adoring patients, watched me and waited.

A slow wave of recognition began. "What is 'this,' exactly?"

He nodded. "This is medicine, man."

To see why physicians are famously bad at understanding and treating pain, at empathizing or listening—at generally tending to human beings—one need only look at the average physician's day in a typical hospital. The day is a flurry of documenting and reviewing numbers, adjusting orders, checking X-rays, and tweaking dosages. A minimum of time is spent on patient contact, and most time that could potentially be used for patient contact is not.

This pattern of patient avoidance is an integral part of a modern medical system that is at least partly responsible for substantial increases in longevity and improved quality of life. But it is also a key contributor to decreasing patient satisfaction and increasing alienation. One of the great secrets of modern health care is, therefore, the lack of care. In hospitals, where virtually all paradigm building and modern training occurs, a tiny fraction of a physician's day is spent seeing, touching, or talking to patients. Physicians learn from the earliest moments of their education that numbers, lab tests, and X-rays are more important. Time spent thinking about these things, time spent reviewing and gathering data, is, in the House, time well spent. Such time is rewarded and affirmed. Time spent on the moments that truly satisfy patients (communication, contact, interaction) is discouraged, forced to compete with the putatively more valuable time spent on numbers, charts, tests, and X-rays.

Over the past two or three decades, physician discontent has increased. Studies indicate that fewer doctors are satisfied with their work, and that increasing numbers are likely to discourage young people from a career in medicine.[1] The impact is felt by all—studies show that dissatisfied physicians are highly associated with dissatisfied patients.[2] In the many physician surveys displaying reasons for this disaffection, at or near the top of the list is the dearth of time spent interacting with patients. We know it, we hate it, and we can't stop doing it.

The fact that physicians want to spend more time with patients, and yet don't, may seem odd. Increasing managed care, overcrowding, and declining federal reimbursements have all contributed to the perception that face-to-face patient time has plummeted over the past twenty years. Physicians complain about being deprived of time with their patients so frequently that in medical circles, the problem is taken for granted. But the most recent and largest study to address average visit times through the 1980s and 1990s found a result that surprised those inside and outside the field: time spent on each patient visit over the past two decades hasn't decreased, it has increased.[3]

Patients seem to want time with physicians, physicians claim they want time with patients, the average amount of time spent together is increasing, and satisfaction among both groups is dropping. Something is wrong, and it's not the amount of time.

———

At 1:53 A.M. Alice awoke in her hospital bed, dizzy. Slowly she reoriented. To her right was a thick white curtain separating her from her "roommate," an empty bed. To her left was a pole that looked like a hat rack, save for a sagging, half-empty bag of intravenous fluid dangling from a peg, dripping quietly. With effort she sat up straight, and the dizziness worsened.

At age fifty-five, Alice considered herself healthy, but for the past week she had noticed blood in the toilet. Two days ago she had seen Dr. Golding, who, in addition to being her primary doctor for years, was a certified gastroenterologist. He examined her in his office, though it seemed perfunctory—he barely touched her, quickly declaring that the problem was hemorrhoids. She was relieved that it was, in his words, "nothing dangerous."

She had followed his directions religiously, using warm baths, but yesterday Alice was surprised by a large painless rush of blood that stained her clothes and furniture. Dizzy, short of breath, and embarrassed, she went to the emergency department, where doctors found her heart rate to be high and her blood counts to be dangerously low. She was told she needed blood transfusions and further tests, and that Dr. Golding would see her in the morning to do a colonoscopy. Maybe it wasn't just hemorrhoids after all.

At 1:55 A.M., two minutes after the dizziness woke her, Alice arose from the bed and walked unsteadily to the bathroom, escorting her IV pole. At 1:56 A.M. a nurse frantically called out for help when she found Alice in the bathroom, semiconscious, in a wall-to-wall pool of blood. Alice remembers seeing the blood, hearing the screaming, and placidly accepting her death.

At 1:57 A.M. the on-call physician was paged. Nurses helped Alice back into her bed, quickly transfused more blood, and rechecked her vital signs every five minutes for the next two hours. Her heart was racing and her blood pressure was low. At 2:13 A.M. a nurse wrote in Alice's chart, "MD paged again, no answer." Alice was now coherent and her color began to return. Still no physician came.

The next entry in her medical chart is at 4:18 A.M., when a physician writes: "Nurses report episode of bleeding. Vital signs noted, currently stable. Will recheck CBC, EKG, type and cross, chest X-ray, monitor vital signs. Awaiting colonoscopy this morning."

A few hours later Dr. Golding performed the colonoscopy, but didn't have time to speak afterward. Alice stayed in the hospital overnight again, and was told by Dr. Golding the next morning, during his five-minute visit on rounds, that the colonoscopy showed hemorrhoids— just as he had suspected. However, it also showed diverticulosis, small sacs that protrude from the wall of the colon and are prone to bleeding. One sack had blood around it, but since there was no active bleeding, he told her, there was nothing to do about it. Her vital signs were correcting nicely, he noted, and the colonoscopy didn't show any major problems like cancer. Her X-rays also looked normal, her fast heart rate was slowing, her EKG seemed fine, and her blood counts had improved. Unfortunately, he didn't have time to answer questions. He added that hopefully, if all her tests were looking better, she would be going home the next day.

Alice stayed overnight again. Her blood was drawn for the eighth time in three days. She still wondered if the problem was the hemorrhoids or the diverticulosis, and she wondered whether or not she was going to bleed again. She didn't know how she would stop this from happening. And she didn't know why she was still dizzy and short of breath. In the morning, Alice was told by a nurse that her blood counts were fine—it was time to go home.

A longtime friend of Alice's asked me to see her in the hospital, and I caught her just before she left. Alice told me about the last few days as I looked through the medical chart, where I found the sterile notations from her near-death experience (and pictures from her colonoscopy neatly pasted in). We spoke for twenty minutes. Despite three days in a hospital under the care of an intestinal disease expert, Alice was deeply confused, and as uninformed about her medical problems as a person can be.

I explained the test findings, and the meaning and definition of hemorrhoids and diverticulosis, and answered her many questions. We discussed the possibility of these problems persisting, the measures she could take to treat her low blood count, the meaning and cause of her dizziness and shortness of breath, the likelihood of serious bleeding, and the danger signs to watch for. Alice, a bright, curious, and reasonable woman, was effusively grateful. It was among the simplest, most rewarding tasks of my day, and the shortest. So why hadn't her doctor done it?

Doctors love tests, perhaps more than they love patients. It is how we are taught—EKGs, X-rays, MRIs, colonoscopies, CAT scans, blood tests, stress tests, cultures, you name it. We believe in the objectivity, utility, and veracity of test results. Alice's blood counts were low, therefore she was admitted and received a transfusion. When she had a nearly fatal bleeding episode, the on-call doctor didn't examine, touch, or even speak to her—he ordered more tests. When a colonoscopy showed a feasible diagnosis, her doctor deemed the mission accomplished. And when her blood counts improved, Alice was dismissed. Tests were the basis for Alice's initial treatment, the methods for her diagnosis, and the benchmarks of success.

In a sense the tests were, at least partly, warranted and useful. The problem, after all, was the bleeding. Tests allowed us to determine that Alice was bleeding, find out why, and gauge the severity. And the possibly lifesaving transfusions and intravenous fluid that she received were given based on these tests. But consider that Alice came to the hospital for three reasons: she was dizzy and short of breath, she was bleeding and didn't know why, and she was afraid it could be dangerous. When she left, her dizziness and shortness of breath were unchanged, the reason for her bleeding was unclear, and her bleeding could still recur and be just as dangerous. While her test results had been specifically noted and addressed, none of the reasons for which Alice had come to the hospital had been.

Modern medicine's dependence on tests is so profound that testing has now become a surrogate for doctoring. Alice wanted doctoring; instead she received testing. The common problem of overtesting and overreliance on tests is also compounded by an even trickier, and even deeper, secret about tests: we don't understand them.

It was a slow afternoon in the cardiology testing lab, and the stress test technician, Jeffrey, a Vietnam vet with a dry wit and a scowl, looked even more bored than I did. So I stripped down to my Skivvies and hopped onto the treadmill. Jeffrey raised an eyebrow over his newspaper. Then, with a happy sneer, he connected me to the EKG wires. After turning a few knobs and punching a few buttons, he threw down the gauntlet: "Bet you can't hit fifteen mets, punk."

"Mets" is an abbreviation for "metabolic equivalents," the stress test machine's measure of how hard the heart is working. A debilitated heart has trouble doing even three mets, while healthy people often do ten or more. Fifteen mets equals serious exercise. "We'll see," I said, and with a flourish I slapped a one-dollar bill on the table. I tried hard to hide my nervousness—which had nothing to do with the bet.

My grandfather died before he was sixty of his fourth heart attack. The thought scared me, and during the last few weeks of my cushy cardiology rotation, I had been plotting a way to pry some lifesaving, or at least life-prolonging, knowledge from my instructors. Who better than a team of cardiologists at a high-powered medical center to tell me how I might avoid my grandfather's fate? And how better to test my heart than a stress test?

With the treadmill on a 30-degree incline and me running at top speed, I reached seventeen mets. Jeffrey must have feared I'd blow a gasket because he dialed it down quickly, bringing me to a walk, then a full stop. Along with my clothing and the folded pages of EKG tracings from the test, he handed me back my dollar.

"Congratulations on sweating like a pig," he said, chuckling, as he went back to his newspaper.

I managed to smile through my panting and heaving, until I looked at the EKG. I hadn't seen too many stress tests that showed obvious heart disease, but mine didn't look right. I dressed quickly and took the EKG.

Dr. Felder was the first cardiologist I found. Embarrassed to admit it was mine, I told him it was from a twenty-eight-year-old male sent in for a routine premilitary stress test. Dr. Felder took a hard look at the EKG and declared me unfit for duty.

"Why? I mean he's a young guy. Are you sure?"

He nodded his head, ran his hand across the EKG page, and offered his final diagnosis: "Heart disease, plain and simple."

More than a decade later I can look back and say, thankfully, that Dr. Felder was wrong . . . sort of. In part he was right: my EKG tracings were positive for heart disease. But he was wrong too: I didn't have heart disease. This common paradox is difficult to understand, but only because of our preconceived notions about medical tests. Tests are very often wrong.

The Reverend Thomas Bayes, the British son of a Nonconformist minister in the eighteenth century, wasn't a doctor and knew nothing about medical tests. But in 1736 he published a mathematics paper that immortalized him in the world of statistics—and medical tests. In this posthumously published work on the subject of conditional probability, Bayes mathematically proves a concept so fundamental that we all learn it in elementary school: to understand something's meaning, one must understand its context.

For the world of medicine, and for medical testing in particular, Bayes's Theorem means everything. It means that without context, the results of a test have no meaning, no intrinsic truth. In order to derive truth from a test result, the result must be treated as a new piece of information, logically integrated with existing information. In the case of my stress test, the new piece of information was a stress test EKG pattern that is seen in some people with heart disease. The existing information, the context, was that I was a twenty-eight-year-old, marathon-running man with no signs or symptoms of heart disease. Treated alone, the new information could easily lead to a faulty conclusion—that I had heart disease. But put the new information together with the existing information, and the answer becomes far more clear—I didn't have heart disease.

What is striking about this concept is that it means that before I ever got on the treadmill, we knew the answer to my question. Indeed, before a test is performed there's an estimable probability that the person being tested has the disease. Before my stress test one could estimate my probability of heart disease: the chances that a twenty-eight-year-old, healthy, active man has heart disease are roughly one in a thousand, or 0.1 percent.* The stress test is performed, in theory, to determine if I am that one in a thousand. But test results are often wrong; therefore a test result doesn't mean that I do or do not have a disease, it simply indicates an adjustment in the probability. How much of an adjustment depends on both the intrinsic accuracy of the test and the context—who gets tested. In the case of my stress test, the fact that I had such a low chance of having the disease to begin with meant that even with a positive stress test my chances of having heart disease had increased only from one in a thousand to three in a thousand.†

What patients and physicians alike have routinely not understood is that because every test is wrong some of the time, test results don't tell us if a disease is present; they simply indicate when a disease is more or less *likely* than it was before the test result. Stress tests have decent intrinsic accuracy, and therefore a positive result did indicate that it was three times more likely that I had heart disease than an average twenty-eight-year-old. But for someone with a 0.1 percent chance, three times more likely still meant a 99.7 percent chance that I didn't have the disease—that a positive test result was wrong.

The key to getting a result that's correct is the context, or who gets tested. This is the essence of Bayes's point: a test's

---

*By heart disease I mean clinically significant coronary artery disease.[4]

†This calculation is based on combined data on the accuracy of stress testing. The positive likelihood ratio derived from these data is approximately three, therefore the probability of the disease before the test is multiplied by three to arrive at the final probability of disease.[5]

intrinsic accuracy isn't as important as a test's subject. Consider an extreme example: what happens when a man takes a pregnancy test. No matter what the test results say, and no matter how accurate a pregnancy test may normally be, the subject being tested isn't pregnant. Certain hormonal conditions, chemical irregularities in the test strip, and human error can all cause a positive pregnancy result in a man, and even the most intrinsically accurate pregnancy tests will turn positive in nonpregnant people (including men) 1 percent of the time.* But as uncommon as a wrong result may be, it's not as uncommon as a man being pregnant. Therefore before the test was ever done, we knew the answer to whether or not the man was pregnant. The context, who was being tested, was far more important for determining the truth than the test itself. When I mounted the treadmill to take the stress test I was suffering from a common delusion: that the test was more important than the subject. But the problem wasn't the test—it was me.

There are many examples of tests where a positive result is more likely to be wrong than right. Screening tests, tests in people who have no symptoms of disease (mammograms, Pap smears, colonoscopies, and so forth), all have positive test results that are wrong much more often than they're right. With very dangerous diseases, however, it may be worth suffering through the many false-positive test results in order to catch the few with the disease, because it may saves lives. Those who argue for mammograms explicitly embrace this logic—97 percent of positive mammograms are wrong.[7] But while there is strong evidence against mammograms saving lives, the logic for the use of many other screening tests is sound. It appears to hold well for

---

*The tests I refer to here are common home pregnancy tests.[6]

Pap smears for cervical cancer, and stool testing for colon cancer, and perhaps colonoscopies for colon cancer.*

But what about medical tests used for common conditions, where the disease isn't as threatening as cancer? Throat cultures detect the bacteria *Streptococcus pyogenes,* the cause of "strep" throat. Most sore throats are viral infections, therefore physicians use cultures to determine which patients have a strep infection. The problem with throat cultures is that they find too much strep. More than 10 percent of schoolchildren (the group at highest risk for strep throat infections), for instance, have live strep bacteria permanently and harmlessly in their throats,† so even when there is no infection, a culture will be positive. These bacteria create a serious problem, because more than 10 percent of those tested will have results that wrongly suggest strep throat. Physicians live with this, however, because in order to detect strep infections we're willing to tolerate being wrong—some of the time. But how much of the time? Bayes's Theorem becomes critical when we ask this question, because how often the test result will be correct is entirely dependent on who we test. The signs and symptoms of strep throat have been exhaustively studied, and from this research we know that there are four important markers of strep throat infections: tender lymph nodes, fever, visible pus on the tonsils, and absence of a cough. When patients have all four of these characteristics, the chance that they have a strep throat infection is about 50 percent. But when they have zero,

---

*Colonoscopies for colon cancer are as yet unproven but indirect evidence is supportive. In the next few years a few large, important studies will hopefully give us the answer.

†In a World Health Organization review, healthy school-aged children, the group most at risk for strep throat, were found to carry the bacteria between 10 percent and 50 percent of the time.[8]

one, or even two of these characteristics, 10 percent or less will have strep throat.

Imagine what happens when we use the test on a group of schoolchildren that has fewer than three of the four hallmark signs of strep throat. Only 10 percent or less will have a true case of strep throat,* therefore no more than 10 percent of them can have positive test results that are right. But we also know that more than 10 percent of those being tested will have positive test results that are wrong (due to the harmless bacteria in their throat). Therefore, a positive test result in this group is mathematically guaranteed to be wrong more often than right. More positive results will be due to harmless bacteria than due to a strep infection.

This situation, in which a positive test is more likely to be wrong than right, is very undesirable. We perform the throat culture test because we would like to accurately select the patients who should have antibiotics. But when we test people who have a less than 10 percent chance of strep throat, most of the people who are given antibiotics will be taking an unnecessary drug with potentially serious side effects. Unfortunately, the great majority of patients (schoolchildren and otherwise) that have a throat culture have fewer than three of the hallmark signs of strep throat, and often two, one, or even zero. Therefore most people who are given antibiotics because of a positive culture for strep throat don't have strep throat.

Throat cultures are one example of many in which we misuse medical tests, allowing them to lead us to make incorrect

---

*The hallmark signs of strep throat are fever, lymph nodes that are tender and swollen, pus on the tonsils, and the absence of a cough. When someone has all four they have about a 50 percent chance of strep throat. Anything less than four and chances are greater that the throat infection is a virus. This particular number applies to those aged over fourteen, as prevalence changes in different age groups.

diagnoses or undertake worthless or harmful treatments. Stress tests are another. The U.S. Preventive Services Task Force has recommended that people without risk factors for heart disease shouldn't have stress tests, because the test results are so often wrong and lead to further unnecessary tests, or else offer a false sense of security. But every day in this country young people without any risk of heart disease still have stress tests. When we do a stress test on an eighteen-year-old girl, do we gain something valuable? What if it's positive? What if EKG changes occurred that were consistent with heart disease? What would the chances be that she actually has heart disease? Teenaged girls don't have heart disease. Therefore, testing them for heart disease guarantees that any positive test result will be false. The test, like so many others, is a waste of time.

Under the right circumstances some modern medical tests can increase the possibility of accurate diagnosis, and on occasion a test will provide potentially life-saving information. But these occasions arise in a small minority of the tests we perform. That the staple of our culture, the elemental unit of modern medical practice—the medical test—has become a misplaced and often dangerous proxy for real doctoring is one of the most closely protected secrets in the House of Medicine. We have devalued the skills of physical examination, like listening to heart sounds, palpating the abdomen, and performing neurologic examinations. Basic skills like communication and observation have been shunned in favor of testing blood and taking X-rays—tests that take us away from our patients rather than toward them.[9] The decline of these skills is inextricably connected to a deterioration in doctor-patient communication and a drop in satisfaction—the physician with his job, the patient with his physician.

In addition, in our overburdened and costly system of health care, poorly chosen medical testing may represent our most excessive and unnecessary outlay. We want access to the technology and crave the false confidence that tests and machines provide—we believe we can trust in them. The irony is that not only are the tests almost always untrustworthy, they move patients and doctors away from the only real source of trust—one another. Both profess to want more time with the other and yet, robotically, and against all intentions and desires, the patient and doctor move further from each other, and further from the roots of medicine.

The following is an excerpt of a case from the writings of Hippocrates: "Silenus lived on the Broad-way, near the house of Evalcidas. From fatigue, drinking, and unseasonable exercises, he was seized with fever. . . . On the second [day], acute fever, stools more copious, thinner, frothy; urine black, an uncomfortable night, slight delirium. On the third, all the symptoms exacerbated; an oblong distension, of a softish nature, from both sides of the hypochondrium to the navel . . . no sleep at night; much talking, laughing, singing, he could not restrain himself."

Hippocrates' close observations of both the form and the function of the human body seem almost to share the experience of illness. Where today's physicians may visit briefly with their ill patients, Hippocrates' description, like most of his case studies, suggests a seated, contemplative companion, enduring Silenus's illness with him. As for medical tests, Hippocrates used his skills of observation. While today's tests are done *away* from the patient, creating distance, a blood test in ancient Greece meant examining its color, viscosity, and taste. All excretions, all changes in facial expression, all dispositions and emotions, and all bodily evolutions were fanatically observed and described. These were the tests that brought Hippocrates closer to his patient and closer to a diagnosis. Our tests, because of the advanced science that they represent, are often presumed to be more important than their subject, but mathematically and conceptually this is wrong. Long before the Reverend Bayes and modern statistics, Hippocrates understood: the human is more important than the test.

6

WE WON'T UNLEARN

(The Pseudoaxioms)

iley, one of the hospital's best and most composed paramedics, called to me from across the room in an urgent tone.
"Doc, I think you'll want to see this one." He was sweating,
and he and his partner were moving quickly with the stretcher between
them.

I followed them into a room and saw nine-year-old Angel sitting
on the stretcher. His face was a reddish hue and he sat staring
vacantly with his head canted to one side. A trickle of saliva slipped

from the corner of his mouth. As I watched him, Angel lifted his shoulders and took a breath, and a sound like a siren came from his throat, with a second, high-pitched whistling noise behind it. At the strange sound Riley pointed, terrified. "That, that. What the hell is that?"

I yelled to the charge nurse, "Mary, get me help in here and put out an overhead for Peds and Anesthesia!" I moved quickly to cover Angel's mouth with a breathing mask, and began forcing oxygen in. I checked my back pocket for a scalpel.

The nurses arrived while Riley, shaken, told Angel's story. "He's had a sore throat, he saw his doctor. Then, wait . . . then he had trouble breathing about twenty minutes after, after he took the antibiotic. He, um, he wheezed a little on the way in, and then all of a sudden, that . . . that . . . sound. Jesus, Doc, what is that?"

I turned to Pat, a seasoned nurse who was staring at Angel as though he was possessed. "Pat, open the crash cart, give him an IM shot of point-three of epi, then start two lines." She broke from her trance, nodded, and within seconds gave Angel the shot. He didn't flinch.

Mike, one of our senior residents, walked in, saw the mask in my hand, and began setting up equipment for tracheal intubation. Angel made the noise again. Mike stopped and looked at me, anxious. "What the hell was that?"

"It's stridor; it means his airway is closing from the swelling. He's having an allergic reaction. Right now his O_2 saturation isn't too bad, but he'll either get better, and stop making that sound, or in the next few minutes we're gonna be cutting into his neck. You have a scalpel?" Mike shook his head, and I handed him mine. We poured antiseptic on Angel's neck and then watched his oxygen levels on the monitors. The room became a still life except for the rhythmic wail of Angel's breath.

The pediatrician and anesthesiologist arrived, and when they heard Angel's breathing they looked at me, alarmed. "I know, I know," I said. "He got epi, his oxygen is okay, we're waiting. We're hoping."

They nodded, and waited. The anesthesiologist prepared his drugs and equipment, while Mike stood, scalpel in hand, and I squeezed oxygen into Angel's lungs. We listened for silence.

Two minutes passed, and I turned my head and closed my eyes. "I don't think . . ." As if on cue, Angel lifted his hand slowly and tried to pull away the mask. I moved it from his face and found him breathing, quietly.

Angel was suffering from anaphylaxis, a potentially fatal allergic reaction to an antibiotic, but he recovered fully—he was lucky. Estimated to occur once in every four hundred prescriptions,[1] reactions like Angel's are the most common life-threatening side effect of antibiotics, but they're not the only ones. Rare, lethal effects of antibiotics also include liver failure, severe anemia, and toxic epidermal necrolysis (a gruesome condition in which skin blisters and peels away). Fortunately, most people who take antibiotics never have to deal with these potentially fatal complications, though they may suffer from inconvenient ones—diarrhea, rashes, and yeast infections each occur in 5 to 25 percent of those taking antibiotics. In the United States, where antibiotic prescriptions are common, patients are exposed to these risks constantly, and they accept them implicitly. Angel was being treated for strep throat, a disease that leads to nearly 10 million antibiotic prescriptions per year, and therefore twenty-five thousand potentially fatal allergic reactions. This is the cost of treating strep throat with antibiotics, and we accept that cost. But why? Is it worth it? Is it also worth the estimated 1 million cases of diarrhea? Our unspoken acceptance of these consequences suggests that it is. But what if it's not?

In the middle of the twentieth century, at the isolated Francis E. Warren Air Force Base in Wyoming, where the air force performed much of its training through the 1940s and 1950s, a raging epidemic of acute rheumatic fever gripped the military recruits stationed there. Acute rheumatic fever most often occurs sporadically and mysteriously in the weeks following strep throat. In addition to fevers and fatigue, the most common manifestation of rheumatic fever in the Wyoming soldiers was "pancarditis," in which the heart became inflamed and heart murmurs appeared. Rashes and red, swollen joints were also common, and some recruits developed tender, unsightly nodules under the skin of their arms. A small number also developed Sydenham's chorea, or "St. Vitus's dance," a condition named after the patron saint of dancers because of its unique, involuntary jerking movements of the limbs, shoulders, and face. The air force's epidemic was unprecedented: no recorded population ever contracted the condition at the rate of the recruits. In most industrialized populations rheumatic fever is rare, striking fewer than one person in every two hundred thousand. Among the recruits, one in every two hundred was afflicted—for nearly a decade at the base, rheumatic fever became a thousand times more common than normal.

In the weeks during and after strep throat, which is caused by the bacteria *Streptococcus pyogenes,* our immune system reacts to the bacteria by manufacturing millions of custom-made antibodies designed to defeat it should the bacteria ever return. It is a highly efficient technique that normally serves us well, occasionally even conferring lifelong protection (as it does with chicken pox). But in the case of the strep bacteria, for reasons that are unknown, the antibodies we generate can attack our own organs instead, causing acute rheumatic fever. At Warren Air Force Base during the 1940s and 1950s, the recruit population was wracked with a virulent strain of strep throat that was often followed by acute rheumatic fever. Fortunately, as frightening as rheumatic fever can be, it is rarely fatal. It is also transient, usually disappearing from a patient's system forever within a few weeks or months after its onset. Rheumatic heart disease is the exception, for damaged heart valves can linger as a permanent reminder of rheumatic fever.

Until rheumatic fever reached epidemic proportions in the small community at Warren Air Force Base, it had been a difficult disease to study. The military physicians at the base recognized an unusual opportunity and seized it, doing extensive research. In a brilliant sequence of six studies,[2] the physicians used placebos and other modern scientific research techniques to examine the impact of antibiotics on the strep throat infection itself, and also on the rate of rheumatic fever that followed it. They published their landmark results for the first time in 1950, and established definitively that treating strep infections with antibiotics had reduced the chances of developing rheumatic fever. While the antibiotics had little impact on the strep throat itself—which seemed to last equally as long and cause symptoms equally severe—rheumatic fever occurred roughly 1 percent of the time after antibiotics were used. In those patients given placebos, it occurred roughly 2 percent of the time. Using antibiotics had cut the rate of rheumatic fever occurrence in half.

In the early part of the twentieth century, most physicians seeing patients with sore throat had been concerned about diphtheria infections, a major cause of death in children and young adults because of throat swelling that could obstruct the windpipe. While streptococcal infections were common, the fact that they were virtually never fatal and generally abated without treatment led physicians to think of them as a comparatively benign cause for sore throat. But as the air force studies became more widely known, and as diphtheria infections vanished because of an effective vaccine, sore throat treatment began to focus on the prevention of acute rheumatic fever. By the 1960s and 1970s professional medical societies, infectious disease experts, and prominent cardiologists everywhere were routinely recommending that strep throat be treated with antibiotics. Though they still recognized that antibiotics had little effect on the infection itself, a point well documented by the military studies,* the prevention of rheumatic heart disease became the focus of sore throat treatment. This turned out to be an irreversible mistake.

The history of treatment of strep throat and rheumatic fever holds the key to unraveling a profoundly flawed logic that now leads physicians to treat virtually all sore throats with antibiotics. The error is deceptively easy to make, and it happens when we look at the studies from Warren Air Force Base. At the time they were performed, these studies were radical and important. But consider that during history's worst ever epidemic of rheumatic fever, if military recruits were given a placebo instead of penicillin, only 2 percent of strep throats

---

*Large data reviews have determined that antibiotics may have a small impact on symptoms (sixteen hours of symptom reduction out of seven days), although this is no better than basic over-the-counter treatments like ibuprofen and acetaminophen, and is not nearly as good as prescription treatments such as narcotics or steroids. The chance of developing an abscess near the tonsils during the infection may also be slightly reduced, though most who develop abscesses don't show up to a physician until well after the point at which they would have helped. In addition the reduction in the chance of an abscess is so small (affecting fewer than one in every 140 people who have strep throat) and abscesses tend to be so easily managed, that physicians do not typically use antibiotics for this reason.

led to rheumatic fever. Therefore only 2 percent of people with strep throat during the rheumatic fever epidemic, about one in every fifty, could potentially benefit from the antibiotic. The other 98 percent did not contract rheumatic fever regardless of their treatment. In addition, antibiotics didn't eradicate rheumatic fever; they reduced it by half, from 2 percent to 1 percent. Therefore half of the 2 percent who would have contracted rheumatic fever contracted it anyway, even when given the antibiotics. Even at the air force base, during the worst outbreak of rheumatic fever ever recorded, only 1 percent of those taking the antibiotic benefited from it.

What is clear is that antibiotics reduce the chance that someone is going to develop rheumatic fever after strep throat, but only if the person with strep throat was going to develop rheumatic fever. But we don't know who is going to develop it. Therefore the antibiotics' potential helpfulness depends entirely on the chance of rheumatic fever occurring. In the military studies that chance was 2 percent. Today, what are the chances of developing rheumatic fever if you don't take antibiotics?

The air force base was suffering a rate of rheumatic fever that was a thousand times greater than that of most industrialized populations, where rheumatic fever is normally rare. Studies of sore throat in the modern era show this to be truer than ever: in a recent community study with more than thirty thousand throat infections (some treated, some not) there were no cases of rheumatic fever.[3] In the fifty years since the military studies, dozens more sore throat studies have been done with thousands of adults and children. To date, there hasn't been a single case of rheumatic fever recorded in any of these studies, placebo groups included. While researchers at Warren AFB had to treat fifty recruits with strep throat before they were able to impact one of them with antibiotics, today we would likely have to treat more than a million in order to prevent a case of rheumatic fever.*

This changes things. The basis of treatment for any condition is the presumption that the disease poses more danger than the treatment. But 1 million prescriptions for antibiotics (to prevent one case of rheumatic fever) will cause more than twenty-four hundred potentially fatal allergic reactions like Angel's, as well as a hundred thousand cases of diarrhea and a hundred thousand rashes. In addition, long-term rheumatic heart disease is the target that antibiotics aim to prevent, but only a third of rheumatic fever cases result in heart disease. Therefore, the number of antibiotic prescriptions it takes to prevent one heart problem is three times as high as the number it takes to prevent rheumatic fever. To prevent one long-term heart problem it would take 3 million antibiotic prescriptions, and more than seven thousand reactions like Angel's.†

In medicine as in most professions, some principles are axiomatic. Often these principles are taught by well-intentioned elders who

---

*The incidence of rheumatic fever in the study populations, roughly 438 per 100,000, was approximately five thousand times that seen today, according to the most recent data from the CDC, which indicate an incidence of 0.1 per 100,000.[4] Also, in the military studies all strep throat infections were seen by the base physicians, while in practice less than half of sore throats that precede cases of rheumatic fever are seen by a physician. Therefore the air force base physicians were able to treat twice as many rheumatic-fever-causing infections as physicians in common practice. Therefore 5,000 (incidence ratio of the study population to present-day populations) x 2 (double the physician-accessible cases) x 100 (the number of recruits that had to be treated for one of them to benefit) = 1,000,000.

†It is often asked whether the use of antibiotics may have caused the disappearance of rheumatic fever. Rheumatic fever's decline is due to improved hygiene, nutritional factors, decreased population crowding, improving preventive care, and evolutionary changes in the bacterium. The decline in rheumatic fever began well before antibiotics existed, and occurred without any decline in strep throat infections; that is, strep throat is just as common as it ever was—it just doesn't cause rheumatic fever anymore. Antibiotics are therefore not believed to have had a serious impact on this.[5]

were handed the same axioms by their teachers—they're simply passing them along. But in most cases they've never examined the evidence themselves. When I was in medical school, respected instructors taught us that it's beneficial to give antibiotics for strep throat because it prevents rheumatic fever. We listened to this axiom and we believed. Perhaps it was easier to believe than to investigate and confirm, but we didn't have time to scrutinize every axiom we were taught. Unfortunately, had we done the research on this axiom, we would have noted that nobody has ever had rheumatic fever at the rate of the Wyoming soldiers, and then we might have asked: Why are we basing strep throat treatment today on air force recruits from the 1940s? Had we asked this question we might have noticed that antibiotics for strep throat are likely killing far more people than they're saving.

The misuse of antibiotics is distinct from the overuse of antibiotics noted in chapter 2. Antibiotics don't work for ear infections and bronchitis because those infections are overwhelmingly viral. Most physicians know this. They prescribe the antibiotic because it has become an accepted norm for both patients and physicians, and because it seems easier to do so than not to, despite evidence that it doesn't work. In the case of sore throat, however, there are studies to suggest that antibiotics are beneficial (the military studies), and common teaching is that they should be used. In bronchitis, physicians know that antibiotics don't work; in strep throat, physicians have convinced themselves that they do—they have embraced a pseudoaxiom.

When an axiom is handed down from generation to generation and it's false, it is a "pseudoaxiom." Like pseudoscience, pseudoaxioms are false statements masquerading as truth, and in modern medicine they're disturbingly common—as common as strep throat. But medicine isn't the only domain in which medical pseudoaxioms exist. Many have crossed into the lay world, settling comfortably in the minds of the general public. The danger of bladder cancer from saccharin, the perils of knuckle cracking and arthritis, and the potential for developing pneumonia from being exposed to cold weather are all pseudoaxioms. There's no reason to believe that saccharin causes bladder cancer in humans; there's not a shred of evidence that knuckle cracking leads to arthritis; and pneumonia is an infection—it comes from germs, not the weather. These pseudoaxioms, these common myths and misunderstandings, are still handed down as facts from generation to generation.

Persistent, baseless assertions of medical "truth" are common in the lay world. But while it's not surprising to hear of nonexperts trading misinformation, it's deeply unsettling to hear about false science among the elite of medicine. And it's disturbing to think that a problem as common as strep throat is being regularly, and dangerously, mismanaged. Patients don't see their doctors because they're hoping to prevent rheumatic fever. They're in pain and feel ill, and they want it to go away. The strep throat–antibiotic pseudoaxiom has shifted treatment away from what matters—the pain and discomfort—and concentrated it on antibiotics, which we have known for decades to be ineffective for strep infections, and which we now know to be harmful.

A final unsavory detail is, therefore, how we communicate with our patients about the routine prescription of antibiotics for strep throat. Many physicians are under the impression that antibiotics benefit patients because they prevent rheumatic fever, but no physicians tell their patients this. We quietly pretend that we're treating the strep throat—not the rare potential for a secondary disease—and then we implicitly take credit for the patient's inevitable recovery from the strep throat. Angel's mother didn't know that the antibiotics were meant to prevent an exceptionally rare disease that occurs a month *after* the sore throat. Instead she was led to believe that antibiotics were the way to rid Angel of the infection. If she had known the truth, would she have consented?

There are many reasons why we have not yet unlearned the sore throat–antibiotic pseudoaxiom. One is the near universality of the teaching that antibiotics are beneficial. Another is that modern physicians like the idea of treating infections, and we dislike the idea of treating symptoms. Treating a bacterial infection with something designed to kill bacteria feels appealing. Pseudoaxiom or not, it feels right. As an added bonus, it has the same benefit as treating bronchitis with antibiotics—it's quick and easy. Sore throat? No problem, here's a prescription. The physician is on to the next patient, and the sore throat patient seems satisfied. Everybody wins. But everybody loses. The antibiotic serves only to endanger patients and to reinforce a mistaken perception of need, and it leaves them without any treatment for the problem that brought them to the doctor: pain. The undertreatment of pain, however, is a category of pseudoaxiom unto itself.

It surprised me to see Nox, a maximum-security prisoner with tattoos and scars all over, grimace when I lightly touched his abdomen. Like me, he was twenty-eight and grew up in New York City, but our lives were otherwise impossibly different. He had a shaved head, a tattoo that said, "It's All Good," on his massive left biceps, dragon and barbed-wire art across his back, and a large scar from a knife wound in his flank. His hands were cuffed together and one leg was strapped to the bed railing.

Nox and I talked about the Upper West Side back in the day, and the deserted train tracks under Riverside Park, though he had trouble concentrating on the conversation because of the persistent "stabbing" pain in his belly. It occurred to me that of all the patients who had told me that their pain felt like a stabbing, Nox would know.

As a med student considering surgery for a career, I nervously presented Nox's case to the chief surgical resident, who challenged me to commit to a diagnosis. "I'm concerned," I said with feigned confidence. "I think something's going on in his belly; I think he'll need surgery."

The chief resident waved as if there were a fly in his face. "Nah. Looks like nothing. We'll get an X-ray." He added, "Then we'll send him back to his jail cell. Next?"

His confidence impressed me, and I nodded hard enough to give myself whiplash. "Sure, okay, yeah. Probably right." Then I thought about Nox for a moment, and in a meager afterthought offered, "Should we give him some morphine or something for pain?"

The chief resident looked at me as if I had just thrown a quick jab to his chin. "Excuse me?" he asked. "You never, ever give narcotics for abdominal pain until you have a diagnosis. That's how you kill people. Make 'em happy and then we can't tell the difference between needing surgery and needing a lollipop. Got it? Remember it."

I nodded, feeling like a fool, and for the next hour tried to distract Nox with memories and bad jokes, while he writhed.

A few minutes after the X-ray was taken, the radiologist came running out of the back room waving the film in her hand. It showed the evidence of a perforated ulcer that would need immediate surgery. The chief resident nodded as if he'd known all along. And as they rolled him toward the OR, Nox looked at me from across the room, managed a smile, and pointed to the three words tattooed on his left biceps.

In 1921, Dr. Zachary Cope, a British surgeon famous for his bedside teaching, his love of writing, and his passion for medical history, published a textbook entitled *Early Diagnosis of the Acute Abdomen*. Cope's brilliant elucidation of principles to divine the problems roiling unseen in the abdominal cavity made the book an instant classic. Over a dozen revisions later, it remains the definitive and most influential work on the subject. Medical students and surgical residents consider it a staple, referring to it simply as *Cope's*.

In one passage of the first edition, Dr. Cope wrote, "Though it may appear cruel, it is really kind to withhold morphine until one is certain or not that surgical interference is necessary, i.e., until a reasonable diagnosis has been made." Thus one of medical history's most powerful and durable pseudoaxioms was born. To be fair, after more than eighty years of technology and medical evolution, it is miraculous that *any* of the material written in Cope's textbook in 1921 is still relevant or applicable, and yet most of it is, a testament to the author. But Dr. Cope also wrote a number of books other than this famous text, including a biography of Florence Nightingale and several works related to British medical history. His prolific pen, combined with a prolific record of public service, led to Cope's knighthood in 1953, and not long before this Sir Zachary Cope had published what may be his least known and most curious work: *The Diagnosis of the Acute Abdomen in Rhyme*. Another treatise on the diagnostic intricacies and challenges of abdominal disease—but this time, all in couplets. In the following passage Cope discusses diagnostic principles in the case of a gentleman seen during a house call for sudden, severe abdominal pain:

> *The face shows pain quite vitriolic*
> *Which obviously can't be colic,*
> *For patient does not writhe or strain*
> *In effort to escape the pain,*

But lies quite motionless and still
Showing he must be gravely ill
For any slight change of position
Just aggravates his sad condition.

Of the doctor's diagnostic conclusion, Cope says:

And here we may assume the doctor stated
"I think this is an ulcer—perforated—
And to the hospital we now must send
This patient if he's ever going to mend."
The diagnosis made, he gives a dose
Of morphine tartrate, and off the patient goes.

And finally, of the surgeon's findings in the operating room:

A cut is made—free gas is found
Which rushes out with hissing sound
Then floods of gastric contents flow
But soon by suction off they go—
Then one can see the perforation
The cause of all this perturbation.
This is sewn up with all due care
By Lembert's sutures here and there,
And to make this water-tight
Omentum's sewn on to the site.
The wound is sewn up and if luck attends
We may say here the moving drama ends.

The Acute Abdomen in Rhyme, which goes on for hundreds of pages in this bouncy fashion, is an entertaining read for medical and nonmedical types alike, and like its prosaic predecessor it has more than a few useful diagnostic pearls. But of interest in the passage above is Sir Zachary's mention of "morphine tartrate." The name of the drug is not often heard today, since the contemporary version is morphine sulfate, a liquid form designed for injection. In 1953 and before, however, the predominant form of the drug was morphine tartrate, a crystallized version that came in two possible doses: either thirty or sixty milligrams.

This dosage is remarkable given that today morphine is frequently given in *one or two* milligrams per dose. The daring physician may give up to five or in extreme cases ten milligrams,* but never thirty. In fact, most present-day physicians would think it sheer insanity to administer thirty milligrams of morphine all at once, not to mention sixty. While it would certainly extinguish any pain, a thirty-milligram dose would also likely send a patient into an immediate and frighteningly deep sleep, with a marked propensity for forgetting to breathe. Sixty milligrams would be openly homicidal. However, this is how morphine was administered in 1921. To administer morphine at these levels could very well have obscured a diagnosis—or even killed a patient. Considered in this context, Sir Zachary's statement that morphine may be harmful seems eminently reasonable.

Years later morphine was transformed from tartrate to sulfate and physicians have now adopted infinitely more judicious dosing practices. But it was roughly seventy years before a concurrent transition was made in the language of Cope's textbook, and most surgeons seem not to have noticed the change. Patients like Nox sometimes sit in quiet agony for hours or even

---

*Note that all of this depends heavily on a patient's pain level and previous exposure to narcotics. Those chronically taking narcotics for pain may require doses that would be potentially lethal in individuals who are naïve to the drug or have not had it recently.

days at a time. Noting this discrepancy, a pair of British surgeons performed a study in the mid-1980s on nearly three hundred patients with undiagnosed abdominal pain. To one group, they administered narcotic medication, such as morphine, and to another they administered placebo injections. Then they determined if those who had received the narcotics were any more difficult to diagnose, or had worse outcomes, than the placebo group. Their conclusion: administering reasonable doses of narcotics was not only safe, it occasionally made diagnosis *easier*. By calming the pain, physicians were able to divine correct diagnoses because they were able to examine the abdomen more thoroughly, and elicit symptoms more completely. Since the publication of this seminal study, at least nine more studies have come to the same conclusion.[6] Accordingly, Cope's textbook has been updated since the early 1990s, and it now strongly advocates the administration of pain medication for abdominal pain.

Physicians agree, then. Problem solved—right? Yes and no. The abdominal pain pseudoaxiom is a somewhat unique type of pseudoaxiom, in that surgeons are well aware of the studies noted above. They're even aware that later editions of the source have completely revised its original assertion. But they will not relent. The day after Nox went to the operating room, I raised the issue again and, having done some reading on the topic, cited the studies. The chief resident called the studies "crap," and then said, "Ask any of our attending surgeons." In a sense, he was right—like ostriches with their heads in the sand, his teachers, aware of the studies, agreed with him.

The problem isn't that these surgeons are unaware of the evidence, it's that the evidence is simply irrelevant to them. In 1991, in a prescient and sadly telling statement, Sir Zachary Cope's successor and the editor of his book, Dr. William Silen, replaced the morphine pseudoaxiom with the following note about withholding pain medication: "This cruel practice is to be condemned, but I suspect that it will take many generations to eliminate it because the rule has become so firmly ingrained in the minds of physicians." Sixteen years later little has changed.

To say that physicians manage pain badly is trendy (though certainly true), but while loss of empathy is often cited as the cause, the problem runs much deeper than this explanation implies. The problem is systemic. The vision of disease that modern medicine embraces is rooted in a theory of organ-based dysfunction, in which symptoms of illness, such as pain, are presumed to be external signals of a diseased or malfunctioning internal organ. Consider going to an auto mechanic about an unsettling sound coming from the car. How surprised we would be if the mechanic rummaged around under the hood, then shrugged and produced a pair of earplugs and said, "Wear these while you drive." This is how physicians, and surgeons in particular, are often taught to think of pain medicine. Numerous studies (with universally concordant results) should have changed this faulty thinking generations ago, but the pseudoaxiom is stubbornly persistent.

The obstinate, head-in-the-sand stance of physicians in the face of the acknowledged evidence is so frustratingly common that these faux factoids have become known as "ostrich pseudo-axioms." And there are many. In 1944 a popular hand surgery text stated that "epinephrine (adrenaline) should never be injected into a digit because from this gangrene has often resulted."[7] Adrenaline can be a useful addition to numbing medicines, generally enhancing and prolonging their effect. As with other body parts, the mixture can be injected into fingers for minor surgery, but because of the statement above, as a general rule it's almost never used in the fingers. The book's references for the frightening statement are a group of case reports of grisly blistering and, ultimately, losses of a finger after seemingly minor surgery. But many of these original reports plainly spell out that adrenaline wasn't used in the surgery. In the majority of the reports the patients went home from their minor finger surgery and reportedly immersed their finger in boiling boric acid. While this sounds insane, it was a standard postsurgical antiseptic method, and explains the blistering in the case reports. Blistering, rarely present in infections, is a nearly universal feature of severe burns. In most of these cases the fingers were immersed in hot water or boric acid while still anesthetized, and patients were incapable of sensing that they were cooking their fingers until it was much too late. Gangrene had nothing to do with these cases, and to compound the irrelevance, adrenaline had nothing to do with most of the injections.

Nonetheless, since the textbook's readers (and editors) apparently never read these original reports or checked the veracity of the cited references, the statement remained, and it resonated. More than sixty years later the overwhelming majority of physicians still cite the use of adrenaline as a gross and indefensible malfeasance that would be certain to condemn a finger to death. I have seen physicians confronted with these data. I've watched as they are shown the original textbook statement and each of the reports that are cited. Finally, they are shown recent medical literature detailing thousands of safe uses of adrenaline by contemporary hand surgeons (the few that are aware of the complete safety of adrenaline).[8] In the face of this incontrovertible and voluminous evidence, reasonable and intelligent physicians often remain irrationally resolute. Today, this adrenaline pseudoaxiom continues to be taught in medical schools and training programs everywhere. It is a pseudoaxiom for some, and an ostrich pseudoaxiom for others.

• • •

Like everyone, physicians are often dogged about the knowledge they have acquired, and it can be exceedingly uncomfortable to confront the suggestion that they were educated incorrectly. Challenging doctors to treat pain more aggressively, or to refrain from prescribing antibiotics for sore throat, or to utilize adrenaline when anesthetizing a finger, is an affront to their foundational theories of medicine and a rebuke to years of their own practice. With this much at stake, in some cases they not only believe something to be true, they *want* it to be true. And when people want something to be true, facts often become subjugated regardless of the weight of the evidence.

Which brings us to the next pseudoaxiom, perhaps the most publicly circulated and widely accepted pseudoaxiom of the past twenty-five years—the one that everyone wants to be true.

Gerard was a thin teenager with a sideways grin and a dipping swagger that was so exaggerated it looked like a limp. As he entered the classroom where I stood at the chalkboard, he put one hand in the air and announced, "Yo, I ain't touching my balls!"

The room filled with inner-city teenage boys broke out in laughter, screams, and high fives. It was my first class in a series of teaching sessions with local high school boys, conducted at the behest of my medical school dean, on the subject of testicular cancer and testicular self-examination. (The girls had a female med student teaching them about breast exams, cancer, and gynecologic issues, and we were both supposed to use a full hour of time.)

The planned content of the class took about ten minutes (Gerard's concern was heeded—no demonstrations), so I handed out blank index cards and told the students that this was their chance to ask me anything, anonymously. Yes, I said, anything. I promised to read the cards aloud and to answer them to the best of my ability.

The first card was scrawled in capital letters. I read it aloud: "DO YOU BEAT IT?"

After the high fives, dancing, and screaming settled down, I did my best to answer the question that I presumed was truly being asked: I explained that, biologically and physically, masturbation was fine and normal. They were suspicious. "What about your eyesight?" "What about for football players, it's bad, right?" There's nothing physically wrong with it, I told them. Help yourself.

It took a few more minutes of Q&A for me to get to the fifth card, which contained the question that would, it turned out, be a constant. It was the only query that I could depend on regardless of the high school—rich or poor, suburban or urban, big or small. When I read it aloud, the room fell silent and the class looked at me expectantly— except Gerard, who said quietly, "That's right," winking at me as if we were in on this one together. The question on the card was, "Where is the G-spot?"

For the next few minutes I had the room's undivided attention.

In 1982, the world's view of female sexuality was changed. Alice Ladas, Beverly Whipple, and John Perry wrote a book called *The G Spot and Other Discoveries About Human Sexuality*, in which they explained that there's an anatomic location within the vaginal canal that has unparalleled sexual potential, offering hope of nearly automatic and unusually powerful female orgasms when stimulated. They cited studies demonstrating its existence, in particular a 1951 article by Dr. Ernest Grafenberg, a prominent New York City gynecologist. That article, the book's authors maintain, was the first to mention the existence of this ultrasensitive area, so they named their discovery after Dr. Grafenberg.

In sexuality textbooks used in college classes today, the

spot is frequently referred to, often matter-of-factly. And in surveys of professional women during the past twenty years, the great majority have consistently reported believing that they have a G-spot. Given the sea change in conceptions of sexuality and sexual anatomy that came in the wake of the book's publication, it's worth venturing into the scientific papers that the authors cite as proof of their discovery. Axiom or pseudoaxiom?

In 1950, the *International Journal of Sexology* published a paper by Ernest Grafenberg entitled "The Role of Urethra in Female Orgasm." Dr. Grafenberg's primary focus in the paper is "frigidity," a term he uses to refer to some women's inability to reach sexual climax during intercourse, and he discusses what he calls "erotogenic" zones, including the female urethra (the urinary passage from the bladder to the outside). His review of these matters isn't so much a scientific demonstration of any-thing in particular as it is a recounting of personal anecdotes, through which Grafenberg rambles tangentially. One story con-cerns a patient who had inquired repeatedly as to why she was unable to reach orgasm with her husband. The good doctor apparently suggested that a different partner might be helpful in this regard, and he describes a panting phone call that he received late the next night informing him that he had been cor-rect. In the midst of this high-spirited fireside chat one finds his reference to the G-spot when he states, "Hardenberg mentions that nerves have been demonstrated only inside the vagina in the anterior wall, proximate to the base of the clitoris." He goes on to say, "This I can confirm by my own experience of numer-ous women."

One might think that this cryptic statement can't possibly be Grafenberg's entire "demonstration" of the spot, but in fact it is. He never asserts any scientific evidence of the existence of such a spot, instead he simply lends the weight of his personal experience to someone else's claim of the existence of nerves within the vagina. That's it—no further discussion on the topic.* In an ostensibly scientific journal, at bare minimum there should be a citation of some sort, a reference pointing the reader to the paper or some other scientific evidence that supports the proposition that these nerves, or this area, exist. But there's nothing.

This lack of evidence may be generally in keeping with the editorial demands of the *International Journal of Sexology*, which had an apparently unillustrious existence from 1949 to 1951. Regardless, with diligent search of the scientific literature prior to 1950, it's possible to locate the article to which Dr. Grafenberg was referring. Written by a woman from Pennsylvania by the name of Esther Hardenbergh (Grafenberg had misspelled it), it was published just prior to Grafenberg's, also in the *International Journal of Sexology*.

In her article, "The Psychology of Feminine Sex Experience," Ms. Hardenbergh (no degree listed) discusses the results of a survey that she administered to women that queried their state of mind during climax. Her discussion is rife with colorful descriptions, and in her attempts to set the physical stage for the reporting of the survey's results, she notes at one point, "Nerves have been demonstrated inside the vagina only in the area of the anterior wall, proximate to the base of the clitoris." Again, in keeping with the journal's lack of demands, Ms. Hardenbergh refers to no evidence, study, or other literature, so it's left to the reader to spec-

---

*Though he provides no evidence, Grafenberg does claim, in separate, equally chatty passages of the article, that this area and a number of others are distinct "erotogenic" zones. Others include the inside of the urethra itself ("I have seen two girls who had stimulated themselves with hairpins in their urethra") and the ear (specifically, "insertion of the penis into the external orifice of the ear").

ulate why she believed this was so. She doesn't mention it again.*

If the existence of nerves was proven, they could potentially support the theory of a sexual epicenter in that location (any highly sensitive area will need to have nerves). But alas, it is false. Anatomic dissections by various anatomists and experts over nearly two hundred years have as yet revealed no evidence of sensory nerve fibers residing within the vaginal wall.†

The Grafenberg and Hardenbergh papers certainly make for interesting, if farcically unscientific, reading, but it's worth noting that neither was attempting to establish or report a previously undiscovered anatomical finding; the theory of nerves in this area is an incidental mention in both. *The G Spot,* however, cites further "evidence" for the spot's existence: two case reports published thirty years after Grafenberg and Hardenbergh. In the first, a woman with a self-reported history of ejaculatory discharge during climax is examined and found to have what is described as a visible, palpable area that caused a pleasurable sensation when stimulated. In addition, "The area grew approximately 50 percent larger upon stimulation." The report, from the *Journal of Sex Research,* also notes that the examining physician was initially baffled but "later became aware of Grafenberg's [1950] paper and concluded that the area . . . was the Grafenberg spot."

The second case report is a description of the "sexologic" examination of eleven volunteers, for whom "television talk shows were the major recruitment vehicles" and of whom "six claimed to

---

*As an interesting historical note, after supporting Hardenbergh's proposal of the existence of nerves in the area, in a later rewrite of his article Grafenberg took a different tack, saying: "I am sure that the nerves are not needed."[9]

†I know of no demonstration of significant sensory nerves, other than nerve fibers capable of sensing pain, within the interior surfaces of the vaginal wall. Pressure sensations due to stretching and movement of neighboring structures occurs, but this is different from the capacity of the internal surfaces to sense touch and to therefore produce tactile pleasure. Multiple anatomists have examined this question.[10]

be ejaculators." Examiners "found areas similar to other descriptions of the Grafenberg spot in four of the 11 women." To the best of my research, however, at the time of this second case report (circa 1980), there were no "other descriptions," except the one report previous to this one. We must also note that both of the case reports were written by coauthors of *The G Spot,* which would be published a year later and sell millions of copies.[11] To date, some twenty-five years later, no one other than these authors has reported or validated these findings in an independent study, despite the supposed fact that the G-spot area was palpable and visible, easy to both feel and see—not at all difficult to find.*

In the field of sexology there is frequent mention and widespread discussion of the "female prostate," a reference to vestigial tissue that is the embryologic homologue of the male prostate and has been microscopically identified near the female urethra. In a small percentage of women, about 10 percent, this tissue is believed to lie on the frontal vaginal wall.[12] Occasionally researchers have proposed that these tissues may represent erogenous zones, but this has never been scientifically demonstrated—nor has the existence of nerves in these areas. If this area was the G-spot, it might theoretically be present in fewer than 10 percent of women, and it would likely be microscopic, impossible to see or feel.

Still, the G-spot has become society's sexual pseudoaxiom, recycled and handed down as fact from one generation of adolescents and adults to the next, and casually asserted in textbooks and

---

*This point has its controversy as well: in their book the authors concede that the area may be difficult to find. This is strange (and perhaps clever): in the case studies they cite to prove the spot's existence, the area was reportedly physically conspicuous. Because there is no new evidence presented in the book, and because the book did not have to undergo any form of scientific peer review in order to be published (while the cited case studies did), I am referencing the case studies here.

in popular media. The results can be both harmful and long lasting, and have likely left many women anxious about why they haven't discovered the spot in themselves. In the absence of contradictory scientific data and fact, and often in spite of it, pseudoaxioms can achieve an energy and a life of their own, self-propagating among physicians, scientists, and nearly everyone else.

When Gerard posed the question in class that day I demurred and instead explained what I knew—standard female anatomy, which luckily enraptured the room. I explained that the G-spot may or may not exist and attempted to leave it at that, but Gerard caught me after the class and asked what I knew. I was forced to concede that I knew very little, and went back to the medical literature that evening. I wrote Gerard with my findings. Though disappointed, he retained an optimistic view, as we are wont to do when we want something to be true. "It's possible, though," Gerard said.

Dr. Sydney Burwell, the dean of Harvard Medical School from 1935 through 1949, used to tell his students that half of what they learned in medical school would prove to be wrong in ten years. Since the publication of this astute observation,[13] studies have examined the durability and longevity of "facts" in the medical literature and found Burwell's estimate to be remarkably accurate.[14] His statement is now routinely invoked at medical school graduations and widely quoted in reviews of medical education. The incisive brilliance and the lasting relevance of this famous refrain is hard to overstate. Burwell had recognized that much of what is learned in medical school is not fact but interpretation, and that we are the stewards of a science in its infancy. He wanted his students to know that we have a responsibility to stay current, to constantly revise, unlearn, and relearn as science progresses and "facts" evolve.

Were he still alive Burwell might note that physicians still learn that in order to reduce the incidence of rheumatic fever, strep throat should be treated with antibiotics. This "fact" may have been true at Warren Air Force Base in the 1940s, but today the harms of antibiotics far outweigh any benefit. The evidence overwhelmingly proves that it is time to unlearn this lesson. The same is true for the danger of adrenaline in the finger, and for narcotics in abdominal pain. As for the G-spot, there is no credible evidence to support its existence. On the other hand, Gerard might say that absence of evidence is not evidence of absence. He'd have a point; perhaps it's out there somewhere.

Our science is limited. Every day, in the constant absence of evidence, physicians make educated guesses, as we must. There are, however, many areas of medicine in which important questions have reliable and proven answers—and these answers go unheeded. In some cases physicians don't know the evidence that contradicts their practice, having blindly accepted the teachings of their predecessors. And in other cases physicians are well aware of the evidence but obstinately refuse to reexamine their practice and themselves.

Hippocrates, who worked for years to impact and ultimately reform medicine, struggled with resistance to his own attempts to bring about change. In his typically insightful way, Hippocrates once prefaced an essay on human health with an explanation that many of the new and unfamiliar concepts that he would be proposing might be difficult for his colleagues to accept, given what they had been taught: "Most men, when they have already heard one person expounding a subject, refuse to listen to those who discuss it after him, not realizing that it takes the same intelligence to learn what statements are correct, as to make original discoveries."

7

WE'RE MISSING
THE MEANING

(The Placebo Paradox)

"*R*ef" had worked as a professional soccer referee in Europe in the sixties and hadn't answered to any other name since. He was a thin, cantankerous World War II veteran and a throat cancer survivor with a tracheostomy, a permanent scowl, and a practiced evil eye. We knew Ref well in the emergency department, mostly because of his previous bouts with mild pneumonias. But when the ambulance delivered him to us this time, he was fighting for his life. He leaned forward with his hands on his knees, sweating and struggling to breathe. We moved quickly around him as his heart raced and his oxygen levels dropped. The veins in his neck stood out and the muscles between his ribs sucked inward with every breath, a primal effort to help his lungs move air. We gave him oxygen mixed with aerosolized medicine through a mask, started an IV, and rapidly took an X-ray. After struggling like this for twenty minutes with no signs of improvement, Ref's breathing abruptly paused. He was ashen and dripping with sweat, and I prepared for the worst. He leaned back, turned to the ceiling, and became perfectly still for a moment. He then heaved forward powerfully, hacking an inch-thick ball of mucus from the hole in his neck. The respiratory therapist turned and threw up into the garbage. After this, Ref lay back on the bed with a wicked grin and breathed freely. His color returned and his vital signs were soon back to normal. The mucus had been plugging his trachea, suffocating him. The emergency was over.

Stunned silence filled the room until Janet, a nurse, yelled, "Good one, Ref!" Within a few minutes Ref collected himself and reinstated his scowl, though I thought this time there was a hint of irony in it.

Minutes later the radiologist called us urgently to inform us that Ref's X-ray showed signs of intestinal rupture. Puzzled, I went to his room, felt his soft and nontender abdomen, confirmed that he was feeling fine, and then examined the X-ray. Believing it was an error, I reordered an X-ray. The next one looked the same. Baffled, we consulted the surgical team, hoping we had misunderstood. The surgical team evaluated Ref and informed us and him that he would need immediate surgery to fix his ruptured intestine.

Ref looked at the surgeons and sneered. He refused the surgery.

As a junior resident, I remained silent while attending physicians debated back and forth. The surgeon conferred with the radiologist, who reconfirmed his reading. Ref scowled anew with each physician's *approach. As a last-ditch measure, the surgeon consulted the on-call psychiatrist, who deemed Ref incompetent. They took him to surgery against his will. Ref shook his head obstinately as he was rolled to the OR. I tried to reassure him. "You'll be all right, Ref, you've been through worse."*

In the operating room the surgeons discovered that his intestines were normal, no rupture. A portion of Ref's colon was resting atop the liver, an unusual situation that on X-rays can falsely mimic a ruptured intestine. Ref recovered slowly, with a difficult bout of pneumonia in the ICU. I wished I had stood up for him.

I saw Ref two months later with his caretaker at a clinic appointment, and against all the rules I apologized, profusely. He scowled. His caretaker told me that he had been eating better since the surgery and that he had repeatedly told her that he felt better; he believed the surgery had worked. Before he left, Ref beckoned to me. In his whispery voice he said, "Thanks, kid." Again, I wondered if there was a hint of irony in it.

I have always felt that I made an error the day I allowed Ref to be taken to surgery against his wishes. He was drugged, his body invaded by tubes and wires, and he was sliced open and his insides manipulated. A strong case for kidnapping and assault could be made. And yet Ref felt that the surgery helped him. Nothing was done in the operating room that could have improved anything for Ref. In fact, he nearly died from pneumonia, a complication of the surgery. So why was he feeling better?

In 2002 an unusual study from Houston's VA Medical Center was published. It was a study about surgery for osteoarthritis of the knee, a condition that causes pain and disability due to thinning and breakdown of cartilage (the padding) in the joint. Patients occasionally have surgery to shave off the rough edges of the cartilage, or sometimes to "wash out" the knee joint. There were three groups of patients in the VA study: one group got the cartilage in their knees shaved, another group got their knees washed out, and one got an elaborate act. When the patient arrived in the operating room he was given anesthetic and the surgeon was then handed a sealed envelope telling him which surgery to perform. If the card inside the envelope said "placebo," three incisions were made in the skin but nothing surgical was done to the knee joint. In case the patient was able to subconsciously hear or feel, water was "splashed to simulate the sounds" of the surgical procedure. In addition, the patient was kept in the operating room for the length of an actual surgery, during which "the surgeon asked for all instruments and manipulated the knee" as if surgery was being done. The operating room staff was sworn to secrecy, and outside the operating room no one was told which surgery the patient had undergone.[1]

The study results were shocking to many, including the orthopedic physicians who perform knee surgeries every day: the two real surgeries had been no more effective than the sham surgery. In retrospect, perhaps this should not have been surprising. Osteoarthritis is due to thinning of the knee cartilage, and there never was a good or even very feasible argument for why either of the treatments, shaving or washing, should work; after all, neither cures or reverses the thinning. But what is surprising even in retrospect is that all of the groups showed significant improvement in knee pain and function. In an article about the study and a closely related smaller study by the same researchers, one gentleman who had been enrolled told an interviewer that he was now able to mow his lawn and walk wherever he wanted, and added, "The surgery was two years ago and the knee has never bothered me since. It's just like my other knee now."[2] He was in the placebo surgery group.

Whether or not the placebo effect is real is a long-standing debate. Judging from this study, it is very real indeed. Osteoarthritis is a serious and progressive disease, and the placebo surgery was a transformative event for many of the patients who had it. The placebo surgery was also at least as good as two of the (still) most common surgeries done for the disease. But some have argued that this study was a fluke. Maybe knee pain is so subjective that results can be manipulated psychologically, with persuasion. Everyone's knees hurt sometimes, it seems. What about a study on something less subjective, on an organ that is deeper inside and harder to manipulate with expectation or persuasion? How about the human heart?

In the late 1930s, cardiac surgeons developed an innovative procedure to help those suffering from repeated chest pains due to severely blocked coronary arteries. The surgery consisted of making two incisions in the chest wall to tie off two unnecessary arteries that supply blood to the inside walls of the chest. Theoretically this could shunt extra blood flow back to the heart, thereby increasing flow through the heart's arteries and reducing chest pain. Initial reports indicated it was highly effective, and case studies showed success rates of up to 75 percent. For the next two decades the surgery became common, until the late 1950s, when two researchers studied the procedure separately and found strikingly similar results. The studies compared the surgery to a sham (placebo) procedure in which two incisions were made in the chest wall and then sutured without tying off the internal arteries. The studies showed the real surgery to be as successful as surgeons had believed. In the true surgery groups, 67 percent of patients showed major reductions in pain and in the need for medicine, and major improvements in the ability to exercise without serious chest pain. But the sham surgery was an even bigger hit: in the sham group 83 percent of patients showed the same improvements.[3]

Subsequent investigations revealed that the artery theory on which the surgery was based was flawed—there's no direct blood vessel connection between heart's arteries and the tied-off arteries, so blocking them would have no reason to increase blood flow to the heart. Why, then, for years, did the true surgery work? Perhaps because the placebo effect is real—so real that it can function viscerally, improving blood flow to an ailing heart. Or maybe there's a more scientifically "rational" explanation: exercise tolerance and pain are subjective, and they depend on effort, and on outlook. Maybe this is another case of psychological manipulation. Perhaps, as some have argued, there is no true physical impact from a placebo procedure, and the real difference in these studies has been the way patients perceive or report their symptoms. Like walking over burning coals, perhaps placebo procedures allowed these patients to overcome their fears, their pain, and the psychological limitations so often associated with illness.

To satisfy the skeptics we must study something that can be measured less subjectively, a disease or organ that depends less on effort or pain and whose physical impact is profound, and can be seen and measured. For instance, Parkinson's disease. Parkinson's, a condition in which a small area in the brain produces progressively less and less of the neurotransmitter dopamine, causes physical manifestations that can be readily measured. Progressive tremors, walking difficulties, problems eating and swallowing, trouble forming facial expressions, and global loss of fine motor control all occur with Parkinson's and are not typically prone to variation based on perception or effort. In addition, the very characteristic that makes Parkinson's the toughest possible challenge for any therapy, placebo or real, is a characteristic that also makes Parkinson's so difficult for patients: the disease rarely if ever improves. It simply progresses, slowly or quickly.

In 2001 a group anchored by Dr. Curt Freed at the University of Colorado published the results of a remarkable study that was the product of well over a decade of experimentation. Dr. Freed is among a handful of researchers who believed for many years that brain cells from human embryos implanted into the small area of the brain that produces dopamine might help to stimulate production of the neurotransmitter, thereby improving the physical manifestations of Parkinson's. Dr. Freed performed a trial based on this theory with a real and a sham surgery group. Because brain surgery is dangerous, the study population was rigidly restricted to Parkinson's patients who were no longer improving with any medications—only those who were rapidly and relentlessly progressing, and failing to respond to all other therapies, were allowed to participate.[4]

The surgery worked. The improvements in patients' ability to perform daily tasks, their quality of life, and their motor function were most pronounced in the first four months following the surgeries. In this case, the true surgery group showed more improvement than the sham surgery group, which means the transplantation technique may hold real promise. But just as notably, those who received the placebo surgery had also improved, this time under the most unlikely and difficult of circumstances. The inevitable question was raised: Can the placebo effect have increased a diseased brain's dopamine production?

Just five months after Dr. Freed's group published their work, a group in Vancouver, Canada, published a study that answered the question. Using a brain imaging technique called "positron emission tomography scans," or PET scans, the researchers recorded the production of dopamine from the diseased areas of the brains of Parkinson's patients. While this had been done before, the researchers performed the images on an unusual group: patients from the active treatment and placebo groups of a trial being done to test a new drug for Parkinson's at their medical center. The PET scans showed that patients receiving placebos had visibly and measurably increased dopamine output from the diseased cells. The PET scans had allowed researchers for the first time to *see* the placebo effect.[5]

Ben was a local television news anchor. His normally well-tanned face was pale, and he was sweating profusely, gritting his teeth and holding his left side. He writhed on the bed, searching for a comfortable position, and told me that he felt as if someone had punched him in the back when he wasn't looking.

"What the hell is it? What's going on?" he asked.

"Looks like you've got a kidney stone, Ben."

"Okay, great," he said through his teeth. "Now what?"

I put my hand on his shoulder and looked him in the eye while a nurse put an IV in his arm. "You're about to feel better, Ben. We've got a lot more pain medicine than you have pain, so don't worry. We know how to make this pain go away."

Ben nodded, put his head down, and took a deep breath. When he looked up again less than a minute later, his color was back. He looked at the IV and saw the fluid dripping into his vein. He looked at me. "You're right, Doc, it's already better."

I didn't tell him that the IV was water, and that he hadn't yet received the pain medicine.

Though placebo surgeries provide stark and intriguing evidence of the placebo effect, studies of the placebo's application to pain, and symptoms such as nausea and sedation, offer consistent examples of placebo effects that researchers can readily study. Many revealing and notable facts about the placebo effect have been gleaned from placebo research:[6]

- Two pills are better than one. Pain is relieved more by taking two placebos than one, and more stimulant or sedative effects occur with two placebo pills than one.
- In one headache study, a placebo pill reduced pain. But with the brand name of a well-advertised aspirin product printed on it, the same placebo pill reduced significantly more pain. Even better than that was a real aspirin pill with no markings on it, and best of all was the same real aspirin pill—with the well-advertised brand name printed on it.
- In the United States, needle injection placebos are more effective than placebo pills in relieving pain. In England, however, there seems to be little difference between pills and injections. But even in England, both provide significant relief.
- Placebo back-pain machines that emit sounds and have blinking lights when attached to patients are more effective at relieving pain than treatment by a physician.
- When given specific expectations, patients connected to placebo machines commonly "feel" an electrical current that isn't present. Patients occasionally volunteered that it felt "just amazing."
- "Nocebo" effects are common. These are adverse effects suffered by patients taking placebos, and include reactions such as facial swelling, rash, dizziness, dry mouth, nausea, diarrhea, and a variety of other symptoms.
- Pink or red placebo pills tend to have stimulant effects,

while blue placebo pills tend to act as sedatives. Both occasionally produce "relatively severe" reactions.

- An antidote that reverses the effects of narcotic pain medications has also been found to reverse the pain relief offered by placebos.

Let's review the last bullet point, one that baffled researchers for quite some time. A medicine called naloxone, a narcotic antidote, is used to treat narcotic overdoses. It works rapidly to reverse the effects of narcotic medications, immediately waking up unconscious overdose patients and also bringing back any pain that was relieved by a narcotic. Remarkably, when a patient's pain has been relieved by a placebo, giving naloxone can reverse this placebo effect. Researchers eventually concluded that naloxone had this effect because of the existence of internal pain-relief substances that are released by the brain and act like narcotics. They're called endorphins, and they were discovered largely because experiments with placebos demonstrated that they must exist. When Ben's pain began to improve, partly because I told him that it would and partly because he saw and felt fluids entering his vein, he was sensing the pain relief and euphoria that come from endorphins—his own body's endogenous narcotics.

It's difficult not to snicker at some of these facts. A beeping machine with lights—"just amazing"? But behind the levity lies a common misconception about the placebo effect: that it's a purely psychological artifact, or a sign of suggestibility. The notion that placebos are a sort of practical joke, and that those who fall for the joke are gullible, is a misconception that has been proven wrong repeatedly. Studies have attempted, unsuccessfully, to identify a personality type, or a telling characteristic, that defines a person who will respond to placebo, but it turns out that we're all "placebo responders." However, the existence and degree of a placebo effect depends on many things. There's a component of conditioning, as with Pavlov's dogs. We associate a pill or an injection or a brand name with pain relief, so nerves are stimulated, biochemical changes occur, internal substances are released, and pain is relieved. There's also a component of expectation. We expect pain relief, and we fulfill our own expectations through internal mechanisms like endorphins. Other components play a part as well, including the desire for healing, the doctor-patient bond, confidence in the physician, and so on. But all of these factors depend on a central and indispensable feature: perception.

Strange proof of the role of perception in the placebo effect comes from the field of acupuncture, and a spot on the arm called the Neiguan. On the inner forearm near the wrist, this spot, also known by acupuncturists as "P6," has been used for hundreds of years as an acupuncture remedy area for nausea and vomiting. In studies comparing P6 acupuncture with a sham (using a needle in an area considered to be inactive, or using a sham device that gives one only the sensation of a needle insertion at the P6 spot), acupuncture at the P6 location, either before or after the surgery, is highly effective in reducing postoperative nausea and vomiting. The effect, however, is seen only when the acupuncture is performed before or after anesthesia, i.e., when the patient is awake. When the acupuncture needle is inserted while the patient is unconscious, it is ineffective. The impact of this acupuncture procedure is entirely dependent on the patient's perception of the procedure. But the true acupuncture provides significantly more relief than a placebo (sham) acupuncture, therefore there is a "real" physiologic impact of the procedure. The correct physiologic stimulus must be combined with perception of that stimulus for a person to experience the impact.

Skeptics have argued that these studies don't provide evidence of a true physiologic placebo effect because pain, or even nausea, can be a subjective measurement. But dopamine output in the brain, and endorphins, are not subjective. Physical healing is also not subjective. Just as more pain reduction is seen with two placebo pills than with one, ulcers seen by endoscopy in the lining of the stomach or intestine heal more quickly when a patient is given two placebo pills rather than one. "Real" medicine reduces high blood pressure, but an inert pill does so as well, albeit somewhat less effectively. "Real" medications for asthma dilate the lung passages, making it easier to breathe; but if you tell an asthma patient that he's going to receive a medication that will dilate his lung passages, and then give him an inhaled placebo, his lung passages dilate.

The patterns of placebo response are virtually identical to the patterns seen when using an effective pill or treatment with an active ingredient. One study of a cholesterol-lowering medication showed that those who took the real medication survived longer than those who took the placebo pills—the active medicine worked. In addition, those who faithfully took the real medication survived longer than those who occasionally missed doses. But those who faithfully took a placebo also survived more often than those who missed placebo doses. And perhaps most remarkably, the survival rate was better among those who faithfully took placebos than among those who occasionally missed doses but were taking the real medication.

Modern medicine's difficulty in accepting the existence and importance of the placebo effect is rooted in a philosophical debate. Unlike Hippocrates' vision of medicine—as a science for addressing the complete mind-body organism—modern Western medicine has embraced a Cartesian model, in which mind and body are separate. In this model the body is a complicated machine with organs and blood vessels and nerves, and its functions are cause-and-effect mechanisms controlled by the brain. The brain in turn is a complex computer that regulates these body parts and their functions, which are separate from mind, or psychological functions like higher thinking and complex reasoning. These processes take place on a different plane that is physiologically distinct from the function of organs or blood vessels or nerves. However, the placebo effect does not respect this mind-body separation. Recognition of the placebo effect demands a broader view, one that sees perception and other psychological, or mind, processes as affecting and being affected by internal physical functions. While the Cartesian model has in some ways served us well, it has made the placebo effect difficult for us to understand. It has also made some of the simplest diseases we know seem like mysteries, and some of our most effective cures seem like miracles.

Layla was twelve weeks old and as many pounds. Since leaving the Baghdad hospital where she was birthed in a dirty room by an untrained nurse's helper, she had fed poorly and gained almost no weight. I met her under the tents of an improvised hospital, surrounded by wounded and battered casualties of war. She was wrinkled and dry and silent. Her little heart lifted her ribs at what seemed like a thousand times a minute, and her eyes were as dark as wishing wells.

Her father, one of our translators, explained that the staccatos of gunfire, the rumble of tanks, and the smell of smoke were ever-present at their dank apartment. The three families that lived there feared for their lives, and they often kept Layla in a dark corner where they felt she was safest. They didn't have running water or electricity, and because they were often ill they rarely held her, for fear of exposing her to disease. When she arrived at our hospital her reflexes were slow, the level of salt in her blood was dangerously high, and her kidneys were failing.

She spent two weeks with us under warm lights and warmer stares. She was the star of everyone's show, every nurse's favorite. They held her and cooed at her constantly. Her parents sat with her all night, feeding and kissing her, and all the battle-hardened physicians came to "examine" her each morning. After two weeks Layla had gained eight pounds, a shine to her skin, and a hundred friends. Her kidneys were perfect, and she gurgled and pointed and smiled and grabbed. And her eyes were still full of wishes.

Layla was suffering from a condition pediatricians call "failure to thrive." The symptoms include poor weight gain, stunted development and growth, susceptibility to infection, and unexplained organ failure. Studies of children with failure to thrive have demonstrated, among other things, decreased blood levels of growth hormones. Failure to thrive is a common diagnosis among children of severely broken homes, the neglected and abused, and the poverty stricken. But modern science can't figure out why.

No good scientific or medical explanation exists for this phenomenon. Failure to thrive is a poorly disguised alias for "we-don't-have-a-clue-why-this-happens." The affliction doesn't result from malnutrition, infection, physical trauma, or any other single physical process that science has identified. It simply happens when a child doesn't have a sufficiently loving, nurturing environment. But we know, for example, that in the setting of epidemics, war, and genocide, when a mother dies her children become far more likely to succumb as well. If love and affection and nurturing are restored, children with failure to thrive almost inevitably recover. Is this the placebo effect? It hardly seems right to call it that, since inert pills are nowhere in the equation.

In his book *Meaning, Medicine, and the "Placebo Effect,"* anthropologist Daniel Moerman argues convincingly that the "placebo effect" is a misnomer, and is widely misunderstood. The book describes literally dozens of studies that challenge widely held views of the placebo effect. One of Moerman's most interesting and persuasive arguments relates to the critical ingredient in the placebo dynamic—the doctor.

Moerman describes a study in which placebo injections for pain are given to two sets of patients under nearly identical circumstances. In the first, the physician is told that there's no chance that a "real" narcotic medication will be given. In the second, the physician is told that there's a chance that the patient will receive a narcotic. In both cases the patient receives a placebo, but the placebo is far more effective in relieving pain in the second case, when the physician believes that a narcotic may be in the injection. While the impact is very different in these cases, the only difference is in the physician's beliefs.

Layla is no different from any of us. At twelve weeks old she was certainly not "suggestible," or a "placebo responder." She is a human, with a social, familial, and biological context, and she is emotionally and physiologically subject to that context. The only things that changed to bring about Layla's recovery were her surroundings and her parents' behavior toward her. What really changed, what really healed Layla, was their loving contact. Her parents were Layla's healers. Layla sensed their contact and it changed everything, including her mind, her brain, her skin, and her kidneys. There is no mystery here when we understand that the experience of the mind deeply affects the human machine to which it is connected. The mind and the body are not separate.

. . .

Understanding the reality and the depth of the placebo effect, understanding that it's far more than we've previously understood it to be, and finally, understanding that the healer (family, physician, acupuncturist, and so forth) is often the most important dial on the placebo panel—*this* is the foundation that allows us to understand modern medicine's placebo secret. For the secret isn't that we're surrounded by a world of placebo effects, and that we see, use, and depend on them every day. It's also not that the placebo effect is a biologically real and formidable force. The secret is more complicated. The secret is that we denigrate and dismiss the placebo effect, and yet we enlist and even crave it when it's convenient to do so. We want the placebo effect, without the placebo.

A year after a beautiful and windy wedding on a Rhode Island pier, and a few weeks after starting a promising new job, Jess sat quietly with her husband, Mark, waiting to hear the results of the operation for her breast cancer.

At thirty-four years old and in what she assumed was perfect health, Jess had gone for an annual checkup and her doctor had found a lump in her breast. Concerned, the gynecologist sent Jess for a mammogram the same day. As she was about to leave the radiologist's office, the radiologist emerged hurriedly from the reading room in the back and stopped Jess to tell her she needed to find a surgeon, immediately. That day, Jess's morning and evening were lifetimes apart.

Soon after, a biopsy confirmed the lump was cancer, and surgery, a "lumpectomy," was performed. The aim was to remove as much of the cancer as possible, and also to find out if it had spread to the lymph nodes. If it had, that would mean a longer and potentially more dangerous and difficult course of chemotherapy than if the cancer had not

yet spread. In the best case, the surgery would show that no areas
around the lump and no lymph nodes had cancer. In the worst case, the
surgery would show that all of the neighboring lymph nodes had
cancer.

When the surgeon entered the room, he smiled and announced that
he had good news—the areas around the lump were clear, and only
one-third of the lymph nodes had cancer.

The language and culture that surround cancer are often discouraging and frightening.* In everyday language we use the
descriptor "like a cancer" to characterize something as insidious
and destructive. Prominent authorities in the field of cancer
management have advocated a physician approach that empha-
sizes explicitly positive communications with cancer patients.
The positive approach is most likely the one that Jess's surgeon
was taking the day he delivered the news about her surgery. He
was setting the stage for a belief in cure; he was creating expectation, recruiting conditioning, investing in will and desire, and
creating a bond. In other words, he was deliberately enlisting a
placebo effect. Some might call it unethical.

Prior to World War II, physicians everywhere used placebos.
The erudite and well-known Harvard medical school professor
Richard Cabot spoke of "placebos, bread pills, water subcuta-
neously, and other devices" during a speech at the Academy of
Medicine in New York in 1903. He went on to say, "I doubt if

---

*Note the use of the mammogram in this anecdote about Jess. The use of mammo-
grams to help better define the characteristics of a lump is very reasonable. But this
"diagnostic mammography" is a completely different animal than "screening mammography." In medicine the term "screening" means testing people who have no
signs or symptoms. The studies that have shown that the addition of mammograms
to standard care does not save lives are all studies on screening mammography.

there is a physician in this room who has not used them and used them pretty often."[7] As late as 1954, a prominent medical journal published an article openly supportive of the use of placebos in clinical practice.[8]

After World War II, however, medicine and medical research changed profoundly. Partly because of advances in scientific method and partly because of the horrors of the Nazi experiments revealed at Nuremberg, research began to emphasize methods designed to value autonomy, and to neutralize bias. "Double-blinded" techniques, in which both researcher and subject are unaware of which treatment is being used, became standard. Placebos became the accepted comparison for new treatments. For the first time, simply asserting the efficacy of a drug became inadequate; the drug had to be "more effective than placebo." In clinical medicine, a new emphasis on informed consent and a new valuation of patient autonomy were embraced. Paternalism became not only passé but unethical, and placebos in medical practice were impugned as prominent symbols of a paternalist ethic. But not everyone was prepared to cast aside the placebo forever.

In 1961 Henry Beecher, a distinguished Harvard professor and researcher of the placebo effect, published a paper comparing sham heart surgeries in two groups of patients from two different studies (the paper discussed only those who had received shams, not the real surgeries).* Using observations of interactions between the physicians and patients Beecher described the surgeons as "enthusiasts" or "skeptics" based on their attitude toward the procedure and toward the patients having the procedure. Patients of the enthusiast surgeons achieved nearly four

---

*This was the same placebo surgery noted earlier, in which chest incisions were made and then sewn back together, on patients with heart disease.

times more complete relief of their chest pain and heart problems than patients of the skeptics.[9]

If this enthusiasm is truly capable of improving outcomes, was it unethical for Jess's surgeon to present the results of her surgery as positive? He presented the facts honestly, he hid nothing from her, and he implied that the glass was half full. Henry Beecher would almost certainly have called him an enthusiast. But where in the interaction does this enthusiasm lie? Is it in the smile? The body language? The words? What transforms a patient-doctor interaction into one that can help patients to heal?

Miss West, a fifty-five-year-old urban dweller, was sweating, and she held her left hand to her chest over a cross around her neck. "I'm sorry, Doc, I just can't get rid of it." She gasped as she spoke, and shook her head. "Oh my. Panic indeed."

She told me her first "panic attack" happened seven years ago, and they had come almost once a month since then, though they weren't usually this bad. "Does your heart feel like it's racing?" I asked. She nodded. "Short of breath?" Nod. "Feel like you're going to die?" Vigorous nod. "Well," I said, "you're not." I looked her in the eye. "That's why you're here. Nothing bad is going to happen while you're here. We won't let it."

She squeezed my hand.

"Miss West, has anybody ever told you what a panic attack is?"

She nodded and waved me off. "Yes, yes, I know, Doc. I'm anxious, I'm panicky, I know. I've heard it all. But I'll tell you, I never feel anxious before it happens. Like today, I'm watching TV, and bam! Off to the races."

"Miss West, if I may . . ." She shrugged and looked away. I explained to her that "panic" was a misnomer and panic attacks a

mystery, that we really don't know the cause. I explained that panic and anxiety often have nothing to do with it, that there are neurotransmitters that fire for reasons we don't understand, even in calm, healthy, normal people, causing what we call panic attacks. But we just don't know why.

She turned and looked at me for a few moments like I was crazy, and then she started to cry. She held her cross and said, "Nobody ever told me that. Nobody ever told me it wasn't my fault." Her heart rate and breathing were back to normal. "I've tried medicines, and therapy, and . . . everything. I'm so glad to know I'm not crazy." She sighed. "I think God sent me here today."

I saw Miss West about six months later. She stopped in to tell me she hadn't had a panic attack since her visit.

When a cancer patient undergoes chemotherapy and the cancer worsens or doesn't improve, physicians and other health-care providers often say, "The patient failed chemotherapy." It's standard lingo, but an odd way of framing the outcome. The patient didn't fail anything. "Chemotherapy failed the patient" would be far more accurate, but that's not what we say. Subtle semantics like this are remnants of a medical culture that blamed patients for problems like treatment failure, or conditions that couldn't be diagnosed or understood. This outdated sensibility is still ingrained in medical education and professional language, and continues to plague us in our everyday interaction with patients. There are dozens of examples, and "panic attack" is one of them.

While it's true that reducing stress can decrease and sometimes even eliminate panic attacks, the disease isn't caused by stress, or panic. Reducing stress also improves heart problems, helps to heal ulcers, and decreases the frequency of simple infections like colds and bronchitis, but it doesn't cause those either.

Panic attacks are a disease, we don't know what causes them—but we do know it's not panic. In Miss West's case, learning that she wasn't responsible for her panic attacks changed her life. For seven years she had fumbled with a cluttered key ring, unable to find the key to the door that would stop her attacks. Discovering that there was no such key allowed her to walk right through it instead.

In his book, Daniel Moerman calls this phenomenon "Diagnosis Is Treatment." He notes that even when a condition can't be cured or repaired, recognizing its existence is meaningful and potentially therapeutic. Moerman also discusses research that has demonstrated an association between an increasing sense of control and decreased suffering. The term "panic" implies weakness and loss of control, even cowardice. When Miss West understood that we were as baffled as she was, she no longer felt that she was a coward, or that she had weakly abdicated control or "panicked"—she understood that she had a disease. She stopped blaming herself.

Language both reflects and guides how we think, and often determines our effect on others. Using the term "panic attack" is accusatory. For Miss West, it caused what Daniel Moerman would call a "meaning response."[10] Moerman believes that response to placebos and to sham surgeries and to nurturing occur because the brain ascribes *meaning* to ingesting pills or undergoing surgery or being nurtured. This meaning often translates to biochemical and immune system changes that result in healing. And in an elegant example of physiologic parity, it was meaningful for Miss West to realize that "panic" was the wrong word. She had another meaning response to this discovery, only this time it was a beneficial one—she stopped having attacks.

The term "panic attack" is similar to the term "placebo effect," in that both are misplaced and misunderstood. The Latin meaning of *placebo*—"I shall please"—doesn't fit its use, or the way laypeople think of it. The way most physicians understand it is also wrong. When diseased cells in the brain produce dopamine, when Ref feels renewed, when Ben's pain softens, when Layla recovers from organ failure, when Miss West's panic attacks remit, and when Jess's surgeon elevates her confidence in a cure, these aren't "placebo effects." They're biologic and physiologic responses to meaningful events. They are meaning responses. For Ref the meaning was in the travails of major surgery, while for Ben there was meaning in the knowledge that his pain would soon be gone and his treatment had begun. For Layla, the touch and embrace of her parents meant that her life and health were worth having. In Miss West's case the path to meaning was understanding that the language of her illness was wrong—she was not a coward. And for Jess, the surgeon was betting that the path to meaning was hopefulness, and a genuine belief that she was on the right path.

The placebo effect is a specific type of meaning response: the meaning that comes from the ritual of administering and ingesting a pill. Administering an inert pill, however, is always an attempt to deceive. But there's nothing deceptive in suggesting that Layla's parents hold her and sing to her. Between these two ends of the spectrum is an ethical divide that modern medicine seeks to find and mark, and perhaps the simplest boundary is the best: a treatment is ethical when the one administering or prescribing it is honest, open, and believes in its potential healing power. The difference between using a placebo and ethically recruiting the meaning response is therefore in the presence or absence of honesty.

In other parts of this book I've argued that antibiotics "don't work" for bronchitis or sore throat, when compared to placebo.

But what about a meaning response? While antibiotics are no more effective than placebo pills, what if you compare antibiotic pills to nothing? In this case they may be very effective in reducing symptoms or duration. If this is true, then why not prescribe them? Many physicians do this every day. The choice seems more humane than prescribing nothing, and it's certainly easier than resisting patients who request or desire antibiotics. Placebos may be unethical, but it seems unethical *not* to use something that heals.

This quandary, this placebo paradox, leads to millions of prescriptions for not only antibiotics but also drugs for pain, heart problems, depression, ADHD, sexual dysfunction, anxiety, and countless ailments. Every condition has its pill. Pills are the great symbol of our advanced technology and brilliant science. In our culture of modern medicine, there's profound meaning in this symbol. Patients crave our technology, and physicians, the ostensibly objective scientists, take the chance to dispense their powerful science. The magic pill is a quick and easy fix requiring little time and even less effort. That physicians often want to prescribe pills is a secret that runs deep. A physician may think, "This bronchitis sufferer is a smoker," or that the symptoms have lasted "too long," or that "the fever is too high." Though evidence shows that none of these characteristics make antibiotics worthwhile, the doctor will write this in the patient's chart, and he will believe in it. He will convince himself. And when the physician is an enthusiast who helps the patient to believe, the result is powerful meaning.

In the final analysis, however, the line between placebo and meaning is a simple one: truthfulness in the interaction. Antibiotics are proven to be no better than placebo pills for bronchitis—and even though the physician who prescribes them knows this, he won't tell his patient. A quiet deception. In the end, we may as well be handing patients an inert pill and all the deceptions, moral compromises, and long-term harms that come with it.

Wearing a particular sneaker brand can make people feel like they're running faster, and indeed they may be. A specific aspirin product is "the one you trust," and it relieves more pain with that slogan on it. A cough syrup is labeled a "proven" cough suppressant, and therefore for some it is. In studies, the soft drink 7UP tastes better when it's in a green can.

Powerful signs of physicians' confidence and expertise, including the white coat, a soothing voice, an empathetic nod, invoke similar meaning. It's been argued that some fields of alternative medicine depend largely—perhaps even entirely—on meaning responses.[11] If so, are we to conclude that these methods don't heal? Speak to migraine sufferers who see an acupuncturist for their headaches. They neither know nor care that a recent trial found acupuncture for migraines "no better than placebo." In the trial, while acupuncture was no better than a placebo procedure, both were far better than being in the group assigned to the "waiting list," where patients never had contact with an acupuncturist.[12] Many migraine sufferers, and many acupuncturists, have found that the headaches are reduced by acupuncture, and they believe it strongly; therefore, they're right.*

---

*There is a tricky division that I have made here between an acupuncturist who believes in his acupuncture despite research, whom I accept, and the allopathic physician who I say should not be prescribing antibiotics, also because of research. The difference is, I believe, in the care provider: while modern allopathic physicians have been trained to believe in modern research methods and results, my sense is that modern acupuncturists more often neither follow nor necessarily believe in the results of Western research methods as mechanisms to evaluate their techniques. Those acupuncturists who do follow and believe such literature would be just as culpable should they continue to provide therapy in the belief that it doesn't work.

Whether it is the ritual of administering the procedure or the biologic impact of the acupuncture that provides relief is in many ways immaterial to the patients. They just want the pain to go away. But it is a question that helps us immensely in understanding where healing comes from. In such cases, is the healing in a needle? In the case of knee surgery, was it in the scalpel? For reducing a headache, was it in the pill, or on the pill's label? For Parkinson's, was it in the saline drops placed in the brain? The answer to these questions is not magical. It is intuitive: The healing is in the psychosocial and biologic context—the contact, the ceremony, the bond between doctor and patient. The healing is not in the pill or the scalpel any more than the strength to run faster was in the sneaker, or the taste was in the color of the can.

This discovery tells us something important about the placebo paradox in, for instance, bronchitis. Giving antibiotics as a placebo is deceptive and therefore unethical, and in addition they have serious and common side effects and increase antibiotic resistance—they come with a heavy price. But tending to each other, listening, and doctoring comes at no price except time, and a paradigm shift. For patients, speaking with the doctor about what bronchitis is, where it comes from, and what to expect is a meaningful and healing act.

Medical education, taught primarily by physicians, is a reflection of medical culture. Currently, we don't routinely teach the meaning response. In heart disease and major depression, to name only two, estimations of the effect of placebo pills have shown that they're proportionally more effective than most "real" medications.[13] But as a medical student I was taught about the unfortunate necessity of placebo in research, the lowly control group who got only placebo (poor bastards). I was also taught about the dishonesty of using placebos in practice. But the meaning response and the placebo were never separated—in fact, most physicians are unaware of such a thing as a meaning response or a placebo effect, and others deny their existence or dismiss them. It doesn't fit the science that we were taught. But while we may not admit it aloud, inside we know, because when there's little else to do, when all else has failed, we'll prescribe a pill. We deny or dismiss the placebo and yet we invoke the placebo effect. We're trapped in a daily dishonesty. We're trapped by our education, trapped by the undue pressures of our system, and trapped by our desire to heal in a culture of the magic pill.

We can understand and acknowledge the meaning response, and we can separate it from the placebo effect. Placebos deceive, insidiously eroding our bond and quietly diminishing real medicine. Meaning, on the other hand, can heal wounds, cure disease, and save lives. In Richard Cabot's 1903 lecture to the Academy of Medicine on truth and placebos, he said, "The majority of placebos are given because we believe the patient will not be satisfied without them. He has learned to expect a medicine for every symptom . . . but who taught him to expect a medicine for every symptom? . . . It is we physicians who are responsible for perpetuating false ideas about disease and its cure." Cabot concluded his lecture by saying, "I have not yet found any case in which a lie does not do more harm than good . . . The technic of truth telling is sometimes difficult, perhaps more difficult than the technic of lying, but its results make it worth acquiring."

The truth about bronchitis, and failure to thrive, and Parkinson's, and panic attacks, and heart disease is that without deception we can help a person to heal. Though Hippocrates may not have known it, the meaning response was likely the core of his practice, and by all accounts his patients loved and revered him. He was a master healer.

8

YOU'RE A NUMBER

(The "NNT")

*O*n a beautiful August day, the medical student Adam and I
were lamenting not being able to breathe in the glorious air
outside when a woman burst through the emergency department doors.

"PLEASE, PLEASE, SOMEBODY HELP ROSA! SOMEBODY
HELP MY DAUGHTER!"

We ran outside. Across the street was a cab with its driver sitting
quietly at the wheel as though nothing important were happening.

Spilling out of the backseat, unconscious, was eighteen-year-old Rosa. From across the street she appeared dead, though when we arrived at her side we could hear a muffled grunt and see her chin inch forward every few seconds as she tried to breathe.

I pushed forward firmly on the back of her jaw to open her airway, and spoke to her mother as we lifted her into a wheelchair. "Ma'am, is she choking, or . . . ?"

She screamed at the top of her lungs, inches from my face, "ASTHMA! OH GOD PLEASE SHE'S DYING!"

We rolled Rosa inside and began to rhythmically squeeze oxygen into her lungs. Her heart was beating at less than ten times per minute. We placed a tube in her trachea, forced her lungs open with oxygen, started an intravenous line, and watched closely to see whether her heart would recover.

Over the next five minutes Rosa's young heart and lungs began to rebound. She spent a single night in the ICU, and in the morning was up and about, talking and laughing. Rosa was back in school two days later, breathing freely on two new medicines for her asthma.

Nearly a year later, I was speaking to a middle-aged woman, cautiously remarking that we had seen her four times in two weeks for her back pain, and had admitted her into the hospital each time.

"So much pain, Doctor. Can't you tell me what's wrong? Please, can't you help me?"

"I would love to, Ms. Feliz, I just don't know what to do. You've been through this four times in two weeks and we haven't found anything that we can fix, or anything to explain your pain. I'm afraid we don't have much more to offer besides pain medicine."

The woman looked at me closely. Tears welled up in her eyes, and she took my hand gently. "You saved my daughter, Doctor. Do you remember?"

I hadn't recognized her, but she was Rosa's mother. She began to cry. "Thank you, Doctor, thank you. You saved Rosa. Thank you for Rosa."

———

Success and failure in the House of Medicine are occasionally found side by side. Rosa is alive today, and it is largely because of what modern science could do for her critical condition. But we have comparatively little to offer her mother. Their juxtaposition says a great deal about where modern medicine is likely to have its highest impact, and where it is likely to have little or no effect. Although we seldom discuss it, physicians are well aware that there are conditions and diseases for which modern medicine can be of immense benefit, and many others for which our toolbox is nearly empty. One way to understand who we can help the most, like Rosa, and who we can help the least, like her mother, is a simple statistical concept called the "Number Needed to Treat," or for short, the "NNT." The NNT measures the impact of a medicine or therapy by estimating the *number* of patients that *need* to be *treated* in order to have an impact on one person. The concept is statistical: we know that not everyone is helped by a medicine or intervention—some benefit, some are harmed, and some are unaffected—but the NNT can tell us exactly how many.

To understand the NNT, first imagine a hypothetical heart attack treatment called StopAttack. Imagine that 75 percent of heart attack victims given StopAttack survive, but only 25 percent survive if they're not given StopAttack, as shown in the graph. While this is a major reduction in deaths, and would prove StopAttack to be an excellent and effective medicine, note that 25 percent of people will die whether they are given Stop-Attack or not (the bottom portion of the graph) and 25 percent will survive whether they are given StopAttack or not (the top portion). These two groups are both unaffected by StopAttack, therefore the treatment neither helped nor hurt them. For the 50 percent in the middle, however, StopAttack was a lifesaver.

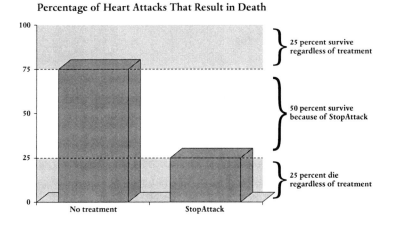

Percentage of Heart Attacks That Result in Death

If we use StopAttack regularly we'll need to treat two people for every one that is positively affected. This number is derived from the graph above, which shows that StopAttack positively affected 50 percent, but didn't help either the 25 percent who would have died regardless of treatment or the 25 percent who would have survived regardless of treatment. Therefore one in two heart attack victims (50 percent) is affected by StopAttack, and there's a 50 percent chance that treatment with StopAttack could save a heart attack victim's life. This means that the number of people we need to treat with StopAttack in order for us to know it affected one person is, on average, two people—the NNT equals *two*.

The NNT is a straightforward way of estimating how likely it is that a treatment or medicine will help an individual person, and the NNT for a drug or intervention is easily calculated from the results of any trial. Since most drugs and interventions have been studied at some point, we know or can estimate an NNT for most drugs or interventions we use, which means that physicians may determine and discuss with their patients the likelihood that they will be helped (or harmed, or unaffected) by a medication or procedure. But as simple as it is to calculate the NNT, for reasons that will become clear, physicians almost never discuss it with patients.

In the weeks before Rosa's severe asthma attack her nights were interrupted by coughing spasms and wheezing, and one mild attack that required an overnight stay in the hospital. She went home the next day breathing easier with increased doses of her medicines. Nearly a week after the hospital stay, Rosa was unable to sleep. She sat up in bed with her inhaler in hand, repeatedly spraying mists of medicine into her lungs to help dilate and relax her airways. As night turned into day her condition grew worse, and the inhaler seemed to help her less and less. In the afternoon Rosa was gripped by a new and unusually strong wave of tightness in her chest, and she began to tire from the seemingly endless work of breathing. Her mother watched as Rosa leaned forward with her hands on her knees, assuming the instinctive "tripod" position of those struggling for breath. Frightened, Ms. Feliz helped her daughter out of the apartment and to the elevator, where Rosa slumped in the corner, exhausted. When they reached the street they found a gypsy cab; in the backseat Rosa closed her eyes and her breathing became more labored. Her mother pleaded with the cabdriver to hurry.

Derived from the Greek *aazein*, "to breathe with the mouth open," or "to pant," the term "asthma" was coined by Hippocrates. Asthma, a disease of chronic inflammation in the linings of the lungs, typically waxes and wanes, and while we know many of the factors that trigger or worsen it, we don't know the cause. The disease may often seem mild and easily controlled, as asthmatics wield their inhalers quietly between sips at the local pub or in the bathroom at a dinner party. But asthma can also be deadly. Rosa was suffering from *status asthmaticus,* a rare and often fatal form of asthma attack. In order to overcome the severe inflammation and narrowing of the airways during *status asthmaticus,* oxygen and medication are forced down the trachea at pressures higher than human lungs can generate, occasionally rupturing and collapsing them. In severe cases, as oxygen levels drop, unconsciousness ensues, and without help, irreversible brain damage soon follows.

The individual NNT for Rosa is a guess, because no one will ever perform a study comparing treatment to no treatment for patients in Rosa's grave condition. Unconscious and in cardiac arrest, Rosa was in the most critical condition possible and required immediate therapy to survive. I would have estimated her chances of survival to be 50 percent. Had we done nothing for her she certainly would have died. Therefore I would estimate the difference between treating Rosa and not treating her to be about 50 percent: 50 percent success if we treated her versus 0 percent success if we didn't. This is equivalent to saying that for every two people we treat with Rosa's condition, one benefits and the other doesn't (one survives and one dies), which means the NNT is two, just as with the hypothetical StopAttack. If, alternatively, only one out of three people in Rosa's condition recovered, then the benefit of treatment would be 33 percent— an NNT of three. If 25 percent survived, then we would need to treat four people in order to benefit one, an NNT of four. And if only 1 percent survived due to treatment, then we would be benefiting only one out of every hundred people we treated, an NNT of one hundred.

The critical point is that the lower the NNT, the more effective the treatment is. The ideal medicine would benefit everybody, and its NNT would equal one—you would need to give it to only one person in order to see a benefit; everyone who receives it benefits. Conversely, the higher the NNT, the less effective and less beneficial the treatment. A very high NNT, say one thousand, means that we need to treat many patients, a thousand, before a treatment will impact even one of them. The other 999 of them receive no benefit.

What's most notable about the NNT is the number of people who don't benefit. In Rosa's case, we're estimating that for every Rosa whose life was saved, one person was treated and didn't benefit—an NNT of two. With a 50 percent chance of being helped, Rosa was exponentially better off than most patients who interact with modern medicine.

The NNT for Rosa's mother is almost infinitely worse. Ms. Feliz had suffered from back pain on and off for years, though it was usually mild, and when she used a heating pad and painkillers it seemed to improve within a few days. But a month before she came to us for her back pain, Ms. Feliz woke up in the middle of the night, unable to find a comfortable position. The pain was radiating into her thighs and wouldn't stop. Her normal measures didn't help, and though her doctor assured her that the pain would decrease, it didn't.

After three hospital visits, an MRI, and a steroid injection (in hopes of reducing any inflammation), the pain returned. As we noted in chapter 1, chronic back pain is a mystery. We don't know where it comes from or how to fix it, and this lack of knowledge translates into an astronomically high NNT. Studies of back pain (surgery vs. no surgery, steroid back injections vs. placebo injections, nerve stimulation vs. bed rest, and so forth) have overwhelmingly produced the same results: no benefit and no difference. In spite of this we can and do treat hordes of people with these interventions, none of which are very effective.

While some individuals may seem to benefit or improve, just as many grow worse, and the great majority are altogether unaffected. Interventions for back pain (other than pain medications) have the highest NNT of all: infinity.

Between treatment for an unconscious girl having a severe asthma attack (among the lowest and best NNTs) and treatment for chronic back pain (the highest and worst) lies a pantheon of modern medical interventions, therapies, and pills. And we know the NNT for these as well.

Already, one woman had chest pain. A new mother wanted to know how much breast milk was too much for her baby. A gentleman had swallowed an insect ("by mistake"). A man had ear pain. A woman felt chills. An elderly lady was in a car accident but felt fine. A child had hit his head on a coffee table. A man wanted to know if kissing transmitted HIV. And there were seven hours left in the night shift.

It was my first night of being on call for a busy family practitioner's office in a small town in upstate New York, and I tried hard to answer everyone's questions. As a medical student doing a rural primary-care rotation, one night a week I was on call for any patients with urgent medical questions. I marveled at the breadth of my ignorance, and the following morning, with notepad in hand, I asked the doctor about each call.

He listened, nodded seriously, and said, "Mm-hmm. Takes a lot of aspirin to get through overnight on-call."

"You're not kidding," I said with a smile. "My head still hurts."

He frowned. "Aspirin for them *is what I meant."*

"What? Like for the car accident lady?"

"Sure." He shrugged. "And the others too."

I shook my head. "Wait a minute—what's aspirin got to do with transmitting HIV?"

"Kid . . . nobody told you this yet? 'Take two and call me in the morning?'"

"Um, yeah. It's a joke, though, right? We don't really say that, do we?"

"Well, not verbatim, of course. But that aspirin is some good stuff." He sat back and took a sip of his coffee.

I looked at him suspiciously. *"What's the point of the other part, then—calling back in the morning?"*

"Now you're getting it," he said. *"By morning most problems are gone. People almost never call back."*

Aspirin may be the most recognizable symbol of modern medical science in all the world. The book *Aspirin: The Remarkable Story of a Wonder Drug* reports that aspirin is responsible for saving the lives of millions and for helping to usher the field of medicine into its modern age. Aspirin is considered one of modern medicine's most useful formulations, and its effects on the human body are well researched and relatively well understood. Aspirin blocks internal chemical reactions that cause inflammation. Inflammation leads to pain, fever, and the activation of platelets; therefore aspirin can reduce pain, fever, and platelet activity. In addition, because platelets are what make up blood clots, the causes of heart attacks and strokes, aspirin also decreases the chances of heart attacks and strokes. Every day, on doctors' orders, tens of millions of people in the United States take an aspirin as a preventive measure for heart attack and stroke. But how much of a wonder drug is it? What's the NNT for aspirin? How many people do we need to treat in order to prevent one person from having a heart attack, stroke, or other vascular problem?

For those at high risk for heart attacks and strokes (those

who are most likely to benefit from aspirin), daily aspirin has no effect on ninety-nine out of a hundred—the NNT for aspirin is about one hundred.[1] In a combined analysis of many studies that together included more than one hundred thousand people at high risk for heart attacks and strokes, researchers calculated that the chance of a stroke, heart attack, or related problem was reduced by 2.5 percent if one took aspirin for over two years. Therefore exactly 2.5 percent of the people on aspirin benefited from it over two years (about 1.25 percent per year).* For everyone else the aspirin made no difference. They were either going to have a heart attack or a stroke, or they weren't.

Percentage Who Suffer a Heart Attack, Stroke, or Death

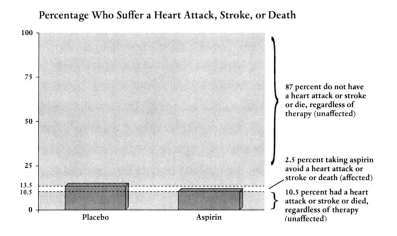

87 percent do not have a heart attack or stroke or die, regardless of therapy (unaffected)

2.5 percent taking aspirin avoid a heart attack or stroke or death (affected)

10.5 percent had a heart attack or stroke or died, regardless of therapy (unaffected)

The graph shows the percentage of people taking aspirin vs. the percentage taking a placebo that will have heart attacks or strokes or die from a vascular problem over a two-year

---

*This is a minor simplification: for some conditions such as heart attack, starting the aspirin in the days after it occurs matters more than in subsequent months, but regardless, because the impact of aspirin depends completely on the prevention of events that we are essentially waiting to happen (strokes, heart attacks, etc.), its total effect is highly dependent on time, or how long one takes it. Every additional year of therapy is an additional opportunity for aspirin to prevent a problem, therefore the total benefit grows every year.

period. In 87 percent there isn't going to be a problem, no matter which pill they take (the top shaded portion of the graph). Another 10.5 percent is going to have one of these problems regardless of the pill they take (the bottom shaded portion of the graph). But 2.5 percent of people will avoid a problem (heart attack or stroke) by taking aspirin rather than placebo. These are the people who are positively affected, at an average of 1.25 percent per year. Therefore, because 1.25 percent is equal to one in every eighty, we have to treat eighty such people with aspirin for one year in order for one of them to benefit—the NNT is eighty. In other words, seventy-nine out of eighty don't benefit from it.

But as striking as these numbers may seem, remember that all medications have side effects—and we haven't yet factored in the chances of hurting someone with aspirin, a critical part of the NNT. In the large research trial noted above there was an increase in the chance of major bleeding, including a potentially fatal brain hemorrhage, among those taking aspirin.* To understand the complete impact of aspirin we have to factor in this serious side effect (which occurred in 0.42 percent more people who were taking aspirin) by subtracting the patients affected from the 2.5 percent who benefit. This reduces the benefit to about 1 percent per year, and increases the NNT from eighty to one hundred. Therefore among these "high-risk" individuals the NNT tells us that ninety-nine out of a hundred people who take aspirin every day for a year will gain nothing from it.

What about the potential benefit for those who aren't at

---

*In the study "major bleeding" meant those requiring blood transfusion or resulting in death. The increase in major bleeding was 0.42 percent. The benefit of aspirin was 2.5 percent, about 1.25 percent per year. This drops the benefit to 2.08 percent and 1.04 percent, or roughly 1 percent, per year.

"high risk"? The patients in the combined analysis above had all been deemed high risk, and indeed the rate of vascular problems like heart attacks in the placebo group was 10.5 percent, an exceptionally high rate. In contrast, an average fifty-four-year-old who hasn't had a heart attack (or similar vascular problem) has only about a 1 percent chance of having a stroke or heart attack each year,* so there is much less opportunity for aspirin to prevent such a problem. For people at this level of baseline risk, aspirin can be expected to reduce risk of a heart attack or stroke by about 0.2 percent over a two-year period,† or 0.1 percent per year. The NNT for the average fifty-four-year-old who hasn't had a heart attack is therefore one thousand. But again, we have to factor in the harmful side effects, which increases the number to 1,176. Though lots of healthy people in their fifties take a daily aspirin on doctors' orders, this NNT means 1,175 out of 1,176 of these people are experiencing no benefit from it.

Why do we prescribe medicines that have a 99 percent chance, or a 99.9 percent chance, of producing no measurable benefit? Because when 1 million high-risk people take this medicine, ten thousand will benefit. And among a million average-risk people, about one thousand will benefit. For each individual the chance of benefit may therefore be exceedingly small, but over large populations aspirin saves lives—and the same can be said for some of the most commonly prescribed pills in modern medicine.

---

*This percentage is an average among all comers. For instance, it goes up if you're a smoker and down if you're not, up if you're a male and down if you're not, etc.[2]

†This number is derived from the original study by using a proportionally equal reduction of risk. In other words, since the high-risk population was reduced from 13 percent baseline risk to 10.5 percent, which is roughly a 20 percent reduction in events, we also estimate a 20 percent relative reduction in risk for other populations. In this case the baseline risk is 1 percent, and 20 percent of 1 is equal to 0.2.

Mindy threw her hands up in resignation. "She's freaking out, Dr. Newman. She insists on getting prescriptions for her blood pressure medicines. I don't do that. What the hell am I supposed to do? I mean, she was here for a few sores on her nose, which I treated, and her blood pressure is normal. But she says she needs to have her medicines. Can you come talk to her?"

Mindy is one of the physician assistants in the emergency department who take care of our less seriously ill and injured patients, treating them for lacerations, fractured ankles, and colds. I spoke to her as I wrote in a chart and looked briefly at a patient's heart monitor. "Well, I'd love to help out, but right now I have my hands full—one guy having a heart attack in Room 18, a teenager with a bleed in his head in 7, and a trauma patient rolling in. So she can wait if she wants, but it'll be a few minutes."

"I bet she'll wait," Mindy said, shaking her head as she walked away. "And she's gonna be yelling at me the whole time."

Half an hour later I walked over to the "FastTrack" area, where Mindy introduced me to Ms. Kern, who was accompanied by her frowning teenaged son. I asked her what we could do for her today.

"Well, Dr. Newman, I am sick today with blood pressure." She emphasized each syllable, and went on to explain angrily that she had not had blood pressure medicines for three months because she had been unable to find the time to get her prescriptions refilled. Now she wanted a new prescription, as she felt her blood pressure was becoming dangerously high.

As delicately as I could, I explained to her that her blood pressure was normal today, and wasn't causing the sores on her nose or any other health problems. I explained that blood pressure is dangerous when it remains elevated for many years, but was certainly not dangerous today, and that she could safely wait to see her physician later in the week.

She pointed at me and declared: "I WILL HAVE MY BLOOD PRESSURE MEDICINES TODAY OR I WILL DIE!"

I offered to call her doctor and arrange an appointment for the very next day, and I tried again to allay her fears by explaining that high blood pressure isn't a disease but a condition that, if it persists for many years, may lead to diseases.

Ms. Kern refused to leave until she had a prescription for blood pressure medication. Surrendering, I wrote her the prescription, and then returned to a room full of emergencies.

Ms. Kern had been conditioned by modern medicine to believe that her (borderline) elevated blood pressure was an immediately life-threatening condition, and that without her medication she might die at any moment. While she was wrong about the urgency,* she may have been correct in her belief that blood pressure medicine could help prevent her from having a serious heart problem. Modern medicine firmly believes in this intervention, and we aggressively treat hypertension (high blood pressure). Of the top ten most commonly prescribed medications in the United States in 2004, six were daily antihypertensives.[3] As with aspirin, the antihypertensives are designed to prevent dangerous heart, kidney, and blood vessel conditions, and as with aspirin, they work.

A large review of the impact of these medications on people

---

*High blood pressure is a condition that increases the chances of developing a dangerous disease like a heart attack. High blood pressure is not the problem. On very rare occasion blood pressure can remain severely elevated for long periods and cause heart or brain problems that are due directly to blood pressure levels, but this is so rare it's like hitting the lottery. Consider, for instance, that when we work out or strain, our blood pressure can easily go into the 200s and even 300s. This is neither dangerous nor bad. Temporarily elevated blood pressure, even for weeks and months, is almost never independently dangerous.

over the age of sixty found that during five years of treatment with antihypertensives (compared to treatment with placebo), the reduction in heart attack, stroke, or related problems was 5 percent, or about 1 percent per year. That means that for each year of taking the medication, 1 percent of patients over the age of sixty will benefit, a yearly NNT of one hundred.* The risk of heart attack, stroke, or death increases substantially with age, so the older one is, the greater the benefit of a medication that may prevent these events, and the lower the NNT. The converse is also true—the younger one is, the smaller the benefit, and the higher the NNT. The data cited above is from a review of elderly patients, therefore the NNTs for everyone else are higher, and less favorable. And as with all medications and interventions, once we incorporate the harms and side effects, the NNT increases and the benefit drops, for all age groups.† In the case of Ms. Kern, in her forties, for every complete year that she faithfully takes her blood pressure medication, the chance is greater than ninety-nine out of a hundred that she'll obtain no benefit from the drugs.

With the NNT as a tool to gauge the potential benefits and harms of an intervention, we can revisit interventions mentioned in earlier chapters, such as mammograms, or antibiotics for strep throat. In the case of mammograms, attempting to calculate the NNT is a misapplication—studies haven't shown a benefit. Because the NNT is derived from whatever the sta-

---

*Again, this is a gross average of the effect over time.[4]

†Many of the serious side effects with these medicines are poorly studied and their incidence disputed. Dangerous electrolyte imbalances, dangerous throat or mouth swelling, and serious heart rhythm disturbances are all well-known problems among the various antihypertensive medicines.

tistically identifiable benefit there is for an intervention, when there is no benefit, there is no NNT. However, the mammogram studies that demonstrated that there is no benefit were only the very high-quality studies. Studies judged to have flaws in their design or problems in the way they were executed were excluded from this analysis, and some mammogram proponents have argued that when we interpret the mammogram data we should include the studies that we know to be flawed because there are a great many of them. They have also argued that we should use "breast cancer mortality" (rather than "overall mortality"—see chapter 2 for an explanation of the difference) as the outcome. If we believed, as these mammogram supporters do, that the mammogram data should be viewed this way, then we can find a benefit to using mammograms in these studies. The benefit that can be found in breast cancer mortality is 0.05 percent, or an NNT of two thousand after ten years of mammograms.

Despite the fact that this is an NNT derived from flawed data and a misleading outcome, we can propose for hypothetical purposes that there is a one in two thousand chance of benefiting during a ten-year period of regular mammograms. With this NNT in mind we can examine and compare the harms that will occur due to ten years of mammograms. An estimated 19 percent of the women who have mammograms will end up having an unnecessary biopsy in this time period, and false positive mammograms, which will occur in about half of all women, will cause severe daily anxiety in roughly 17 percent. Presuming overlap between these two groups, and counting these as the only harmful side effects, an estimated 25 percent of women undergoing mammograms will experience a harmful side effect. From an NNT of two thousand we can see that for every one woman who benefits from a mammogram, five hundred more will suffer severe anxiety or an unnecessary surgical procedure on their breast.*

With strep throat and antibiotics, you will recall that when we calculated the likelihood of preventing rheumatic fever in chapter 6, we determined that we would need to treat roughly 1 million strep throats to prevent a single person from contracting rheumatic fever (NNT of 1 million), because rheumatic fever is rare. Using this number, we can compare the potential harms of antibiotics to the benefit. Antibiotics will cause an estimated 10 percent to have diarrhea; another 10 percent will contract a rash; and approximately 10 percent of women taking antibiotics will suffer a yeast infection. In addition, an estimated 0.24 percent will suffer a life-threatening allergic reaction, and we can estimate that about one out of every ten of these people will die. Therefore, for every one case of rheumatic fever that we prevent by treating 1 million people with antibiotics, we also cause an estimated one hundred thousand cases of diarrhea, one hundred thousand rashes, and one hundred thousand yeast infections. And we kill 240 people.

An analysis using the NNT can help us in determining priorities for other common and recommended medical therapies. The controversial website hospitalcompare.hhs.gov was created by the Centers for Medicare & Medicaid Services, an agency of the U.S. Department of Health and Human Services. The website allows consumers to see how well each hospital performs for the treatment of specific conditions. One can determine, for instance, how often a hospital gave heart attack patients a class

---

*25 percent of 2000 = 500. There are, of course, many other true harms to mammograms that could have been included here but are not, for simplicity.

of drug called "beta blockers" immediately upon arrival at the hospital. Beta blockers slow the heart and reduce the force of its contractions, theoretically calming the heart and reducing damage. Many groups, including the American Heart Association, recommend early administration of beta blocker medications during heart attacks.

When we examine the NNT for beta blockers, however, the evidence for early application isn't so clear. First, the only high-quality studies that have been done on beta blockers have been on patients having major, obvious heart attacks, but most heart attacks are subtle, and less dangerous. Second, for the patients in the studies the calculated NNT is over a hundred, and even this small benefit is still uncertain.* Let's presume, however, that there is indeed a roughly 1 percent benefit of early beta blockers in patients during obvious heart attacks (an NNT of one hundred). You'll recall from chapter 3 that identifying most heart attacks early is tricky because signs, symptoms, EKGs, and blood tests are all unreliable. Generally it takes an overnight stay in the hospital to determine definitively whether or not a heart attack has occurred. But the Hospital Compare website doesn't ask whether or not the heart attack was readily apparent when the patient arrived; it asks only whether beta blockers were given when the patient arrived. However, since we usually don't know whether or not patients were suffering a heart attack until twenty-four hours later, in order for hospitals to achieve high numbers (the website is monitored and reported on by media outlets), hospitals must treat not only those obviously having a heart attack, in

---

*The AHA guidelines[5] cite three studies to support administering beta blockers right away in heart attacks. The reduction in mortality was in the range of 0.7 percent in the two larger studies and 3.2 percent in the smallest and least convincing study.[6] The problem is partly that heart failure and shock seem to be significantly increasing in those receiving beta blockers.

whom one out of a hundred may benefit, but also anyone they think *might* be having a heart attack—and most aren't.

The NNT in this case must therefore be calculated for the use of beta blockers in *possible* heart attacks. Only about one in twenty people being evaluated and treated for a possible heart attack is truly having one.[7] If one in a hundred people who are having a heart attack is benefited by beta blockers, but only one in twenty people is actually having a heart attack, then only one in two thousand people (100 x 20 = NNT of 2,000) is truly benefiting from the drug. The benefit of a drug vanishes when the patient doesn't have the disease that the drug treats—but the risk of suffering a side effect stays exactly the same. According to the *Physicians' Desk Reference,* roughly 3 percent of those treated with beta blockers experience shortness of breath or a dangerously slowed heartbeat, 1 percent suffer a dangerous drop in their blood pressure, and 1 percent develop wheezing and difficulty breathing. Less serious problems (diarrhea and rash) each occur roughly 5 percent of the time.* By adding in these risks to our NNT we can see that for every one person out of two thousand who benefits from beta blockers, a serious, potentially life-threatening side effect will occur in approximately one hundred more people, and a less serious side effect will occur in another two hundred. The drug harms three hundred times more people than it benefits.

A final note on beta blockers for subtle heart attacks. For any medication or therapy, the more serious and life-threatening the condition, the greater the potential benefit. This is simple logic

---

*PDR 2007 data reported for metoprolol (the most commonly used beta blocker in most emergency departments). These side effects have been best documented in patients placed on the medicine for weeks to months, not those receiving a few doses of the medicine. The adverse effects for those receiving first doses in the setting of possible or confirmed heart attacks are less well documented.

manifest in the NNT: if no one dies from a disease, it is impossible for treatment of that disease to prevent death. The more who die or suffer from a disease, the greater the chance of providing a benefit. The NNT of two thousand that we have calculated on the use of beta blockers for subtle heart attacks is therefore certain to be an underestimate. For while it may be argued that a few studies have shown beta blockers to be of benefit in major heart attacks, there is not a single piece of reliable evidence that they're helpful in subtle, rarely fatal ones—the ones we're using them for the most.

As medical technology marches forward, swallowing increasingly large portions of our health-care budget and generating new medications and procedures, the NNT can also shed a critical light on new therapies and technologies, helping us to make reasonable decisions about when and how to use them. In 1999, despite concern expressed by prominent cardiologists, the FDA approved two new pain medications: Vioxx and Celebrex. Within a few years the drugs were blockbusters, with gargantuan profits and tens of millions of annual prescriptions. But five years after their debut, the tides turned. Evidence demonstrated that Vioxx causes a small but significant and consistent increase in heart attacks and vascular problems, and Celebrex does the same. But if a small increase in harmful side effects was enough to bring about their reversal of fortune, what precisely was the benefit? What was the NNT?

The producers of Vioxx (Merck) and Celebrex (initially Pharmacia, now Pfizer) hoped that the medications could partially replace drugs like ibuprofen and naproxen, cheap and effective pain medicines that carry a 1–2 percent risk of serious gastrointestinal side effects. The newer pain medications were members of a class designed to reduce these side effects, and in late 2000, two large studies, one of Celebrex and one of Vioxx, tested their side-effect profiles in comparison to the older drugs. The first trial compared Celebrex to ibuprofen and diclofenac, and reported a difference that was so small that the authors were forced to concede that the new and old drugs were "statistically indistinguishable"—there was no apparent advantage to Celebrex (an infinite NNT). Why, then, did the FDA approve Celebrex, and why did millions of prescriptions follow? Perhaps because instead of dwelling on the drug's failure to achieve its intended goal, the authors instead emphasized that Celebrex "was associated with a lower incidence of symptomatic ulcers and ulcer complications combined." This late change in the study's parameters turned a failure into an apparent success. Though the study was designed to test the drug's effect on ulcer complications alone (and not in combination with any other factor), the authors instead combined ulcer complications with a minor, more subjective, secondary measure—symptoms— which resulted in a better-looking number.* The makers of

---

*The authors had earlier judged symptoms of ulcers to be too unreliable to be a major study end point, choosing instead to measure intestinal rupture and major bleeding as the important end points the study was to assess. This was an appropriate choice both because preventing the more serious outcomes is far more important, and also because, as you'll recall from chapter 1, the symptoms of ulcers are nonspecific and unreliable. Yet after the study was done the researchers combined together "symptomatic ulcers" with the miniscule difference in "ulcer complications." This is misleading. Universally in high-quality studies a single outcome is chosen to determine success or failure of a drug. In the Celebrex study that primary outcome measure was serious ulcer complications like bleeding and rupture, and information on symptoms of ulcers was collected only as a secondary, and noncritical, measure. Studies are designed and built around primary outcome measures, both statistically and methodologically, and no additional secondary data can later determine success or failure of the study drug, even in combinations. These secondary measures are collected so that ideas for future studies can be generated and data can be comprehensively observed, but they are never for determining success or failure. This is because a biased researcher or author could ignore the primary outcomes, instead cherry-picking minor differences that seem to favor their drug, and fusing them until some combination looks major, while ignoring those differences that seem unfavorable.

Celebrex promoted this more favorable-appearing (but utterly insignificant) aspect of the study, garnering excellent press and instant FDA approval while physicians and leaders ignored the infinite NNT, a finding that was there for anyone who cared to notice.

Unfortunately for the researchers, however, an even larger problem soon came to light in a letter to the editor published in the *British Medical Journal*. The letter reported that the study's authors had revealed and submitted only six months of the data from the twelve-month study. When all twelve months of the data were examined, Celebrex looked even worse than it had in the first six months. No sleight of hand could now hide the drug's failure. With new scrutiny, and a new analysis, the infinite NNT became public knowledge.[8] But the FDA had already approved the drug.

The second study, in 2000, compared Vioxx to naproxen and showed a difference that was, incredibly, even smaller than the original Celebrex study had shown.* (This study, like the Celebrex study before it, would also achieve dubious recognition later, as the authors failed to report an increase in heart attacks.[†]) Nonetheless, in an attempt to take the most favorable possible view, if we combine the data from the original Celebrex report with the data from the Vioxx study, we can derive an estimate of

---

*This Vioxx study in the *NEJM* used slightly different definitions of improved outcomes than the Celebrex study published in *JAMA*. The *JAMA* study, however, used outcomes that are universally considered much more clinically important. Therefore I am noting the "benefits," and therefore the NNTs, for the two studies by calculating the clinically important outcomes of ulcer complications. The actual numbers were Celebrex 0.69 percent less ulcer complications, and Vioxx 0.5 percent less ulcer complications.

†The authors of the Vioxx study claim that the original study plan and design precluded them from reporting the heart attacks, due to prespecified time cutoffs for data reporting.[9]

the total difference in effectiveness between the new class of drugs and their competitors—0.61 percent.* Using this, we can calculate an NNT to be, at best, 164. Therefore at least 163 out of 164 people taking the new class of drugs would derive no benefit from them. The NNT makes it possible to tell that with safer, cheaper, time-tested alternatives available on the market, there is virtually no reason to have ever written a prescription for Celebrex or Vioxx.

Why did physicians write prescriptions for Vioxx and Celebrex? The most likely answer is aggressive advertising. Musically catchy advertisements filled the television airwaves in the years following the FDA approval of both Vioxx and Celebrex, and physicians and patients are highly susceptible to such advertisements. A famous survey of British primary care physicians in 2003 demonstrated that physicians frequently use drug sales representatives and advertisements as their primary sources for drug information, rather than the original studies published in scientific journals (from which an NNT could be calculated). Despite this, surveyed physicians felt that free lunches and golf trips did not affect their prescribing behaviors.[10] Literally dozens of studies have shown that individual prescribing patterns are significantly influenced by such tactics,[11] and while surveyed physicians typically do concede that advertising affects both patients and doctors in general,[12] they most often believe themselves immune.

Many factors contributed to the Celebrex/Vioxx debacle.

---

*The number of serious gastrointestinal side effects in the two studies are as follows: Vioxx 16/4047 vs. naproxen 37/4029, and Celebrex 30/3987 vs. ibupr/diclof 58/3981. The combined numbers are 46/8034 vs. 95/8010, or 0.573 percent vs. 1.186 percent. Difference = 0.61 percent. I'll also note here that the Vioxx study reported and calculated more than just "ulcer complications" in their primary end point, but in order to combine apples with apples here I have used only these serious side effects from both studies.

One was the misleading way the study was reported (both in leaving out six months of data, and also in highlighting the less important, but more flattering, statistics), and a second was ineffectual oversight mechanisms.* Physicians individually have no control over any of these factors. But physicians can control the information they seek and how they interpret it. And they can control whether and how they communicate that information to their patients. Had we examined the data ourselves before we wrote a single prescription, and had we calculated and articulated the NNT, everyone would have known from the beginning, long before we found that their harms were greater than their benefits, that Vioxx and Celebrex were born losers.

On July 10, 2002, a *New York Times* headline read, "Hormone Replacement Study a Shock to the Medical System." The article began: "The announcement yesterday that a hormone replacement regimen taken by six million American women did more harm than good was met with puzzlement and disbelief." The article was written in response to the results of the Women's Health Initiative study published in *The Journal of the American Medical Association*.[15] Involving over sixteen thousand women, the study evaluated hormone replacement therapy, a pill regimen that supplements fading estrogen and progesterone levels at the time of menopause. The researchers com-

---

*The FDA has been repeatedly called out for its lack of regulatory power, and also its lack of epidemiology-trained safety personnel involved at higher levels in both drug approval and regulatory oversight. I suspect that the apparent marginalization of these individuals within the agency and in particular in the drug approval process explains how it was that the simple and conspicuous data gimmicks utilized in the Celebrex study were not instantly recognized and the drug denied approval. The Institute of Medicine noted these issues and called for major changes in the FDA,[13] and an *NEJM* editorialist (with past experience working for the FDA) has also spoken out.[14]

pared the hormone pills to placebo pills, blinding both the physicians and patients to which pills they were given. Hormones are known to have a myriad of complicated effects, and for many years conventional medical wisdom held that their replacement (to maintain premenopause levels) might reduce the progression of heart disease. However, the researchers at the Women's Health Initiative feared that hormone replacement might also increase the risk of developing breast cancer, so they closely monitored breast cancer rates among study subjects. If breast cancer increased in the group taking hormones, they planned to intervene (that is, halt the study). To their dismay, after five years of treatment the researchers found that the breast cancer rate was indeed increasing among women on the hormone pills. This result, and the accompanying media coverage of it, caused millions of women to immediately cease hormone therapy.

It is worth revisiting these events with the NNT as a tool. The increase in breast cancers over an average of five years of hormone replacement was 0.08 percent. If we convert this into an NNT, we see that 6,250 women had to be treated with hormone therapy for one year in order for one additional case of breast cancer to result. This means that 99.92 percent of women who took five years of hormone therapy were unaffected by breast cancer. Breast cancer certainly increased with the use of hormone therapy, but with the use of the NNT we can see that the increased risk was small. But there were also increased chances of heart problems, including minor heart attacks, strokes, or blood clots. On the other hand, there were benefits to hormone replacement: a decrease in colorectal cancers and a decrease in hip and back fractures. Finally, a large review by the Cochrane group in 2004 also concluded (from data unrelated to the Women's Health Initiative study) that hormone replacement therapy reduces the frequency of hot flashes by an average of 75 percent.[16]

The many different effects of hormone replacement make understanding their total impact complicated. While the NNT is an excellent tool for understanding the likelihood that an intervention will have an impact in terms of a single outcome like death, or heart attacks, or cancer, it is less helpful when many outcomes may all be affected. To quantify the risks and benefits of hormone replacement therapy we can, however, transform the NNTs into numbers that put the risks and benefits in terms relative to each other: For every ten thousand women taking hormone replacement, there are eight breast cancers *caused* by the pills, and six colorectal cancers *prevented*. In addition, five hip fractures, six back fractures, and 75 percent of all hot flashes will be averted. Finally, seven nonfatal cardiac events, eight strokes (also nonfatal), and eight blood clots will also occur.

This NNT-style comparison for hormone replacement therapy may allow patients to decide if hormone replacement is of use to them individually. In particular, a woman with an average or below average risk of heart problems and breast cancer, but with a concern about—or an elevated risk of—colorectal cancer, or a particular risk of fractures, may decide that hormone replacement therapy is more likely to help than harm her. If hot flashes are an important concern, these too can be factored in. As for women with a particular concern about (or a known risk of) breast cancer or heart disease, they may be comforted to know that even after combining all the cancer and heart disease risks, fewer than one in every three hundred women on hormone replacement for five years will suffer even one of these adverse effects. To put this in perspective, it is far more likely (nearly four times more) that taking a single antibiotic prescription will cause a life-threatening allergic reaction than it is that a year of hormone replacement therapy will threaten one's health.* By comparing NNTs we can see that we have more to fear from a single one-week prescription for antibiotics than we do from five years of hormone replacement therapy.

Finally, an analysis using the NNT for the single outcome of mortality tells us that despite the small increase in breast cancer and heart problems that can develop with hormone replacement therapy, the same number of women in both groups were alive after five years. Despite the well-reported and much discussed risks of hormone replacement therapy, these risks didn't translate into a single additional death out of sixteen thousand women, which makes the distinctions between harm and benefit even blurrier, and the capacity for patients to bring their own values to the decision about hormone replacement even more crucial.

If the NNT is so simple, so powerful, and so useful, why aren't all physicians using it? The simple answer is that they should be, and perhaps some already do in some form. But in reality very few do, and the reasons are complex. One reason is that the NNT reveals truths that are uncomfortable. What the numbers say makes us shift in our seats. We have yet to devise an effective treatment for chronic back pain, therefore the NNT—infinity—is more than a number, it is a message. Few physicians have told their patients that back pain is a mystery to modern medicine. But an infinite NNT does exactly that. The astronomical NNT for antibiotics in strep throat clearly indicates how misguided

---

*Recall that an estimated one in every 410, or 0.24 percent of antibiotic prescriptions results in a life-threatening allergic reaction, while for each complete year of hormone replacement therapy 0.06 percent, or one in every 1,600 women, had a breast cancer or a heart problem in association with the pills.

our approach is. It is easier to avoid these issues than it is to talk about the NNT. A second problem with the NNT is that its educated use requires two mental leaps for the modern physician. The first is acknowledging the placebo effect (and the meaning response), an act that many physicians feel is akin to magical thinking. The second is understanding that the doctor-patient bond may be just as important as any medicine our science has invented.

Recall that in research like the aspirin studies there are two groups: one assigned to take aspirin and a second assigned to take a placebo. The only difference between these groups is the active ingredient inside the pill. Randomization, blinding, and placebo techniques exist for one reason: to maintain perfect equality between the groups—to isolate the "active ingredient" as the only important difference. We do this so that when studies show that a drug "works" we can say that the active ingredient is what worked. The NNT is an estimate of the impact of this active ingredient. But the active ingredient doesn't exist in a vacuum. Both study groups are being seen regularly by physicians, both are counseled on lifestyle issues and treated for illnesses, both are listened to and tended to, and both are given a bottle with pills to take every day. As noted in the last chapter, there is *meaning* in these interactions, with psychosocial context and biophysical consequences. And although the active ingredient can often be important, we know that these encounters can have a significant impact on healing and health. In some cases, this impact is the elephant in the room—somehow unmentioned, and yet bigger than everything else.

Consider the study about acupuncture for the treatment of migraines from the previous chapter. Acupuncture reduced migraines for 51 percent of patients, while sham (placebo) acupuncture reduced migraines by 53 percent. The third group, patients on the waiting list who got no treatment, improved by 15 percent, but those who got acupuncture or a sham improved much more—51 and 53 percent (see graph). Therefore, there was a tremendous benefit to being in these two groups over being on the waiting list. But that benefit wasn't found in the active ingredient (the acupuncture), since the real and the fake acupuncture had the same impact. Instead, the benefit was found in the rituals and encounters surrounding acupuncture. There was a 38 percent improvement among those who were seen by an acupuncturist compared to those on the waiting list (53 percent minus 15 percent), regardless of real or sham acupuncture. That's an NNT of less than three, indicating that the rituals of acupuncture have more impact than some of the most effective active ingredients that modern medicine has ever devised, including aspirin, heart surgery, and some chemotherapies.

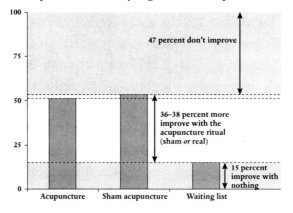

Improvements in Daily Migraine with Acupuncture

The acupuncture study shows an effect on pain, but other outcomes are affected as well. One study examined postoperative swelling and inflammatory blood levels after wisdom tooth extraction. Patients were administered ultrasound or sham ultrasound to the face overlying the surgical area, and in a third group nothing was done to the area. The amount of postoperative facial swelling decreased by 30 percent in both the ultrasound and sham ultrasound groups compared to the no-treatment group. Therefore, while the ultrasound was ineffective when compared to a placebo ultrasound, both were 30 percent better than doing nothing. In addition, the level of "C-reactive protein," a chemical of inflammation found in the blood, had also dropped by an average of 30 percent in the ultrasound groups (both real and sham) when compared to the no-treatment group.[17] Again, the overall effect was an NNT of three, and again, there are few active ingredients in modern medicine that show this level of effectiveness.

These studies indicate that the significance of the tending ritual of patient-doctor contact is real, and so is the response. The actions and interactions of the patient and doctor when acupuncture is performed, the shared experience of tending and communication, had an NNT that was more powerful than that of almost any pill science has produced. While the hard science, the active ingredient, should therefore be respected and given the credit it is due, the NNT also demands that we acknowledge and understand the simplest, and in some cases most powerful, medicine of all: the contact between doctor and patient.

The contrast between the NNT for Ms. Feliz's back pain (infinite) and her daughter's asthma attack (two) tells us about the strengths and weaknesses of modern medicine. In the emergency departments of modern hospitals, we're well equipped to handle immediate threats to life, from heart attacks to gunshot wounds to choking. For these problems the NNT is low. At the moment that someone is choking, the Heimlich maneuver has an excellent NNT. Rather than prevention of a potential problem (an endeavor usually associated with very high NNTs), the

Heimlich maneuver is treatment for an immediate threat, choking. The NNT for daily aspirin is over a thousand for prevention of death due to a future heart attack, but only forty for prevention of death when administered during a heart attack.[18] The pill is the same.

When determining how effective modern medicine (that is, the active ingredient) can be, the sicker one is, the better. Dr. Andrew Weil, the famous proponent of "integrative" and complementary medicine, has called ours a "disease-care" system rather than a health-care system, recognizing that modern medicine is well equipped to care for active diseases but poorly equipped to care for healthy individuals. If a truck hits you, the modern medical system is likely to be of immense benefit, and even Dr. Weil would undoubtedly point his own ambulance to the nearest trauma center. However, if you would like to prevent a second heart attack, Dr. Weil might point out that the single act of quitting smoking is fifty times more effective than twenty years of high blood pressure medicine.

Understanding and appreciating the NNT allows us to understand and choose the preventions and treatments, both collectively and individually, that are right for us. It allows us to understand how modern medicine can benefit us the most. The NNT is not an argument to abandon daily aspirin, or to stop taking medicine for high blood pressure. Large NNTs do not mean interventions have zero value, they simply help us understand risks and benefits. Vaccinations have immense NNTs, but they've saved millions of lives. I wear a seat belt although the chance of my being involved in a potentially fatal automobile accident each time I get in my car is infinitesimally small, far smaller than the chances of a person with high blood pressure having a heart attack. But still I wear my seat belt. It is a calculated decision, one that makes sense to me given what I believe to be the virtually absent downside of wearing it—the adverse effects of seat belts are few and far between. The NNT for wearing my seat belt is therefore extremely high, but well worth it to me, both for my peace of mind and for the real safety it provides.

But the NNTs for medicine have remained the exclusive property of doctors, one of our deepest secrets. The secrecy may literally be killing us. When the FDA approved Celebrex and Vioxx and we ignored the NNT, we paid (and continue to pay) the price in lives. When all women are urged to undergo routine mammograms regardless of the NNT, we're paying the price in mastectomies, biopsies, and the millions of false-positive cancer scares. When beta blockers become a mandatory part of care without an examination of the NNT, we are encouraging our hospitals to harm their patients. When we ignore the NNT for antibiotics in strep throat we put our children and ourselves at serious risk, with virtually no chance of benefit.

The NNT for a drug or intervention is not flawless, and it is not tailored to the individual. It is an average value, not an accurate personal appraisal. And it is possible that medications with high NNTs for outcomes like heart attack and death may provide secondhand benefits, like improved quality of life and daily health, and decreased susceptibility to infection and injury. These outcomes are more difficult to measure and prove in studies. But we should not fear that use of the NNT will be misleading or wrong. We have lived for too long without the NNT, and without any serious disclosure of the impact of our medicine; therefore, even an imperfect tool will bring us far closer to the truth than where we are now.

Hippocrates talked about the virtues and power of the doctor-patient bond: "Some patients, though conscious that their condition is perilous, recover their health simply through their contentment with the good of the physician." Hippocrates believed that his greatest impact was not in his science, but in his presence. He practiced an Art that first and foremost respected his patients, placing them above all other considerations. They were not nameless numbers or a means to an end, and he did not seek to use only the active ingredient. Today we practice an Art that often places method above outcome, science above people. When the NNT from our active ingredient is one hundred, we pursue the benefit of the one at unspoken risk to the ninety-nine, and we quietly pretend that there is benefit for all. This approach has been expensive—personally, professionally, and financially. As we spend hundreds of billions of dollars on measures with NNTs that show them to be conspicuously detrimental, confidence in physicians and science plummets, patient and physician satisfaction declines, and the doctor-patient partnership is increasingly driven by forces like advertising or poorly considered government benchmarks.

But there is hope when one considers the potential in truth, and in transparency. There is, after all, nothing mutually exclusive about acknowledging how large or small a benefit may be, and still reaping it. Our powerful science can work perfectly in concert with our powerful bond. In the past our choices have often ignored the NNT. When we understand that the bond between us is the source of perhaps the lowest and best NNT, and when we prioritize our therapies with the NNT in mind, we'll be that much closer to medicine's ideal, where everyone benefits: an NNT of one.

THE "NUMBER NEEDED TO TREAT" FOR VARIOUS HEALTH-CARE MEASURES, BASED ON HIGH-QUALITY STUDIES

The higher the NNT, the smaller the total benefit; an infinite NNT means no benefit while an NNT of one means everyone using the medication (or intervention) benefits.

Daily aspirin for individuals at high risk (1 year)	100
Daily aspirin for individuals at average risk (1 year)	1,176
Aspirin for preventing death *during* a heart attack	40
High blood pressure medicine for preventing heart problems, over age 60 (1 year)	100
Mammograms, for preventing death overall (high-quality data only, 13 years)	No benefit (∞)
Mammograms, for preventing breast cancer death (high-quality data only, 13 years)	No benefit (∞)
Mammograms, for preventing death overall (low-quality data included, 13 years)	No benefit (∞)
Mammograms, for preventing breast cancer death (low-quality data included, 13 years)	2,000
*Mammograms, for causing a cancer scare (a "false positive"; 10 years)**	2
*Mammograms, for causing a surgical procedure on a noncancerous breast (13 years)**	5
PSA, for preventing death overall or death from prostate cancer[1]	No benefit (∞)
Exercise, for reducing complications of heart disease after a heart attack[2]	37
Lowering salt intake, for preventing heart problems after a heart attack or stroke[3]	42
Quitting smoking, for preventing death or heart attack after a heart attack or stroke[4]	8
*HRT, for causing breast cancer or a nonfatal heart attack**	667
HRT, for preventing colorectal cancer or preventing a hip or back fracture	588
HRT, for prevention of unwanted events (like cancers or fractures) overall	2,000
HRT, for prevention of hot flashes	3
Prayer, for curing or alleviating illness[5]	No benefit (∞)
Celebrex, for preventing a serious gastrointestinal problem	No benefit (∞)
Vioxx, for preventing a serious gastrointestinal problem	200
*Vioxx, for causing a heart attack, stroke, or related event**	59

HRT = hormone replacement therapy

*Measures in italics represent a harmful effect rather than beneficial.

9

A NEW OLD PARADIGM

Somewhere on medicine's path from ancient Greece to the present day, physicians and patients began to drift apart. We have traveled different roads and live in different worlds, and our goals have diverged. Patients come to the House of Medicine to be heard, touched, and understood, and to reap the benefits that they believe modern science offers. Physicians aim to seek pathology and diagnose disease, and to dispense the benefits of science accordingly. Both groups are increasingly unhappy. Patient surveys show that patients feel they lack quality time, communication, and contact with their physician. Physician surveys show that physicians sense a growing and vexing distance from their patients. Both want more of the other, but we are divided by the mistrust and alienation that come from secrecy.

In the House of Medicine, we have been led to believe that our secrets protect both patients and doctors. Patients are shielded from confusion and disenchantment while physicians are protected from the judgment of the uninitiated who they believe cannot understand. Secrets are therefore woven into the fabric of daily medicine: some are subtle and some are conspicuous; some are unconscious and some are deliberate; some are complex and some are simple. But all are costly, as the fundamental goals that physicians share with patients—better health, longer and happier lives, human contact—are being compromised by secrecy. Physicians sense this and it manifests as frustration, "dissatisfaction," and attrition. Overwhelmed by the work at hand and with neither the support, know-how, nor the time to step back for a broad view, doctors tacitly allow these secrets to persist. Physicians are inundated by system pressures, surrounded by peer behaviors, and affected by powerful notions of safety and familiarity. And the nature of secrecy is to spiral. Secrets beget secrets.

The power of the secret is that it separates, locking some in and locking others out. I have attempted to take that power away by offering a beginner's list of secrets doctors keep. These include: our knowledge is far more limited than most believe; we advocate and utilize interventions we know don't work; we disagree on seemingly fundamental issues of science; at system levels we care nothing about communication; we choose technology over touch; we openly defy established evidence; we deny and decry a placebo effect while we tacitly accept and enlist it; and we know precisely how likely each patient is to benefit from an intervention, but seldom tell them.

In the first eight chapters of this book, I have attempted to reveal and explain each of these secrets. This is a first step. But if physicians are to regain our Hippocratic ideals all parties must also understand the larger forces that led to this model of secrecy, as well as the forces that now make physicians feel threatened without it. To accomplish this task we must first discuss the grandest of all threats, the one that induces physicians and patients to withdraw even further from one another. It is the elephant in the room: our broken health-care system.

In the United States we have chosen a health-care system controlled by the invisible hand of market forces. The intent and the hope of such a system is that the population's demand for health care will drive the system to maximize supply until demand is satisfied. The great fear, particularly in a market-based system attempting to provide a fundamental right such as medical care, is that if robust profits are achieved without adequate supply, there is no incentive to improve supply. Has profit trumped supply in our system? The answer is yes: we spent more than $7,000 per person on health care in 2006,[1] the highest in the world by far. In 2004, the most recent year with comparative data, Luxembourg and Switzerland were a distant second and third, spending $5,000 and $4,000, respectively.[2] Yet in common health-care benchmarks (life expectancy, infant mortality, maternal mortality, etc.), we are near the bottom of industrialized nations in virtually every category.[3] Spending (profit) is the highest in the world while performance (supply) is among the lowest. It is not difficult to see whether profit has trumped supply.

In our system, because spending is out of control, it is not profitable to provide private insurance without charging unaffordable rates, which leaves nearly 50 million citizens uninsured. In a telling contrast, however, the procedures, products, and services that generate excellent profits (that is, pills and surgeries) are advertised in lights, often to the exclusion of simpler, more powerful, more advantageous measures. In Atul Gawande's "The Checklist," he details research on a breathtakingly simple method to prevent infections in intensive care units.[4] Physicians, all of whom could recite by heart the proper steps for placing catheters in patients' deep "central" veins, were monitored and asked to verbally follow a checklist of those steps during the procedure. At the study institutions the checklist method nearly eradicated one of the most common and deadly classes of infections in the intensive care units. Yet this remarkable and inexpensive breakthrough is rarely used. Instead, thousands of patients succumb and billions are spent on the antibiotics, personnel, and other resources required to treat the infections. As Gawande points out, if the method were a product, a patented technique, or a pill, it would be in use everywhere. But one cannot generate a special bill, and therefore a profit, for completing a checklist.

The checklist is only one way in which the priority of profit over benefit takes lives. The uninsured and the meagerly insured (those on Medicaid) are almost twice as likely to die after a diagnosis of cancer as the privately insured.* Statistics for established killers such as heart disease and infant mortality are similar.[6] Private insurers brashly exclude those whose need for health care is greatest, because insuring them is not profitable. Lucrative interventions displace beneficial preventive care. It is profitable, for instance, for a hospital and a surgeon to amputate the leg of a diabetic; but it is not profitable to prevent the amputation with high-quality primary care. Amputations are therefore available to anyone (even Medicaid pays for them), while good primary

---

*The risk of death in the first five years after a diagnosis of cancer among the uninsured was 1.6 times the risk for those with private insurance. The number was similar for those on Medicaid compared to the privately insured.[5]

care, a service that could potentially unite patients and doctors, is only for those who can afford it.

In my specialty, emergency medicine, we are besieged by system failures all day, every day. In the past ten years the number of emergency departments has dropped 12 percent while visits have increased 18 percent. Our federal government, whose diminishing aid helped to create the problem, and who mandates that emergency care be provided to all, is now the number-one scofflaw for emergency department bills.[7] But emergency departments remain the one true safety net in our system, loyally and consistently treating each of the one hundred million visitors (one out of every three Americans) that we see each year. The emergency department is therefore an unpaid, and often unprofitable, stepchild in the House of Medicine. We are chronically under-funded, chronically overwhelmed, and in a chronic state of crisis.[8]

Emergency departments are but one piece in our mosaic of failure. Primary care physicians are asked to do more for less and to spend more time on paperwork than on patients. Malpractice costs are rising and lawsuits abound. Physicians order unimportant X-rays to avoid being sued, not because patients will benefit. They order worthless blood tests to mollify those who wait. Slighted patients file lawsuits because their doctor, rushed and disengaged, didn't know their name. Antibiotics are prescribed because it's easy. Important conversations are avoided because of time constraints. It goes on and on.

And yet . . . here we are. While our system's flaws are monumental, our problems are not unique. In health-care systems around the world, profit-driven and otherwise, waiting rooms are full, clinics are crowded, and demand outpaces supply. These are the common realities of providing health care on a large scale anywhere. And while our tattered system exacerbates the problem of our secrecy and our dissatisfaction, it does not create or excuse it. Patients in systems with long waits and limited resources are often satisfied and grateful, while those with shorter waits, better insurance, and more access are often dissatisfied and frustrated.[9] Secrecy and disaffection therefore exist where money is no object, and in highly functional systems, indicating that the most powerful determinant of success or failure is not found in infrastructure but in the point of contact. Our failing health-care system has become an excuse, a scapegoat for our distance and secrecy. The true origin comes from within, at the point of contact, in the bond between patient and doctor. But how? What in our modern mind-set has left us struggling to see and hear each other? What has come between us?

On a brisk autumn evening in 1513, a century before the telescope was invented, a Polish canon and practicing physician, who fancied himself a poet and a painter, gazed at the stars. Astronomy was yet another of his hobbies, but as a former student in the discipline of optics, he took detailed notes. His observations vexed him, appearing as they did to subvert his Christian theology, and to challenge eight hundred years of accepted astronomy. Discreetly, over the months and seasons that followed, Nicolaus Copernicus distributed to friends and colleagues his own *Commentariolus,* a written summary of astronomical recordings and the apparent conclusion they represented. Though eventually he consented to wider dissemination of his work, this came too late to provide the personal recognition it deserved. It is said that on his deathbed Copernicus first held a finished copy of *On the Revolutions,* an unassuming and narrowly technical work that suggested the earth revolves around the sun, rather than vice versa. Man was dethroned from the center of the universe, and the Scientific Revolution was launched.

Although millennia of thought and influence preceded him (and it took Brahe, Kepler, and Galileo to mold his work into an accurate physical theory), Copernicus is widely recognized as having provided the epiphany that would lead our modern world to its love affair with science. We have forged ahead ever since. We now embrace a driving faith that much of the universe is knowable, and we harbor an almost spiritual conviction that what is knowable must indeed be known. In the name of this faith we have invented and innovated tirelessly, and the fruits of our ambition surround us: towering structures, flying machines, pocket-sized devices that link continents, and more. From birth we are awash in the marvels of technology, symbols of the Copernican ascent.

The field of medicine is uniquely positioned within this crusade, for much of our scientific work is done in its name. Medicine offers the tangible impact of science as a weapon against human illness and human mortality, and medical practice and research surge ahead relentlessly with special dispensation, relieved of any responsibility for the moral burden that discovery brings. Medical practitioners and researchers follow in the proud tradition of the great explorers of our physical world who journeyed with an unquestioning faith that exploration is not just a means but also an end, and who did not ponder the meaning of discovery until it was upon them. But in medicine there is profound meaning and urgent context to our discoveries, and the failure of physicians, researchers, and leaders to examine these issues has taken a toll. Inquiries into meaning and context have become the domain of the philosopher and the ethicist, a diminutive pair who, despite a proud history, now trail behind us on our journey, picking up the pieces as best they can.

The ancient Greeks did not ignore meaning in their world. Their conception of technical and physical science included the philosophical arts (they had no word for "science" without "art"). In recent history the philosopher and the ethicist have learned powerful lessons while the rest of the scientific community has largely fixed its gaze on the horizon ahead. Our collective preoccupation with advancing frontiers and our nearly blind faith in science have led us to disregard perhaps the most important philosophic revelations of modern science: those that chart its limits. Great leaps in scientific thought since Copernicus have come in the form of establishing limits, and it is the omission of these from the modern consciousness of both the scientist and the layperson that has crippled medicine. In particular three of these discoveries, though broad in their implications, are ciphers for the origin of our secrecy. They are the discoveries of Bayes, Heisenberg, and Gödel.

Bayes

The Reverend Thomas Bayes was a brilliant mathematician who suffered from a Copernicus-like unease with public scrutiny. The only paper he published during his lifetime challenged the work of a celebrated contemporary, so he published it anonymously. Bayes's greatest work, his only other publication, was released two years after his death by a friend in 1763. The paper was another challenge to an established authority, but this time the authority was far more revered. Bayes challenged the scientific inquiry, the essential element of all scientific exploration, the question that a curious scientist poses to launch the scientific process. It is the elemental unit of the scientific method, the progenitor of all truth. Using the language of conditional probability, Bayes, a practiced mathematician, executed a scientific inquiry into the nature of the scientific inquiry, and in doing so changed the playing field of science. Bayes found that when trying to determine truth, the inquiry and its answer are less important than its context. In chapter 5, I noted the importance of this for medical tests, but it applies to far more. Bayes's Theorem is the mathematical proof that challenges basic presumptions of Western medicine. The Theorem tells us that human health is driven first and foremost by human function and human context.

The statement seems self-evident, yet it flies in the face of modern medicine's daily practice. To illustrate, imagine that a human being is a large panel of buttons, and that each button controls an internal substance, chemical, or function. Though inadequate to represent all human substances and functions, the panel would have one million buttons. To reduce the human's risk of heart disease, one might press a button to decrease cholesterol; to help with anemia or low iron levels, one might press a button to increase iron; to minimize the chance of strokes, one might press a button to decrease clotting factors. This, pressing buttons, is the basic and most common endeavor of modern medicine. But now consider the panel. If the buttons are one inch in diameter and arranged an inch apart, with forty rows, the panel reaches six and a half feet in height and a half mile in length—more than seven football fields long. Bayes's Theorem asks us all, at the moment we press one button, to step back and take in the size of the panel.

In chapter 8, I noted that the NNTs* for many celebrated medications including aspirin and the antihypertensives are strikingly high, often a hundred or more, and in some cases greater than a thousand. The best remedies of modern medicine have NNTs in the range of fifty or, in rare cases, ten. At

*Recall that NNT stands for number needed to treat.

best, tens of individuals, and more often dozens, hundreds, or even thousands, must be treated with a medicine before a single patient has been measurably helped by it. This reality, predicted by Bayes's Theorem, has been largely ignored. Physicians and patients both speak of pills as "miracle drugs," and physicians write and dispense prescriptions as though an individual's life and health depend on them and them alone. But they rarely do. There are limits to what can be achieved by pressing a single button.

Heisenberg

At Niels Bohr's quantum physics laboratories in Copenhagen, a second critical moment in the history of scientific thought came in 1926, when Werner Heisenberg developed the Uncertainty Principle. Like Bayes's discovery, Heisenberg's took both mathematical and philosophical forms, and again the implications were broad. In his investigations of quantum physics, Heisenberg demonstrated that the more precisely a particle's position was determined the less precisely its momentum could be determined, and vice versa. The principle is complex (Einstein struggled with it), but there was a simple deduction: the knowledge that can be gained from observation in the physical sciences is limited in ways that we have yet to grasp. Heisenberg's principle challenged basic understandings of cause and effect and it questioned the applicability and consistency of deductive scientific reasoning to the physical world in which we live.

The House of Medicine, however, continues to treat the human organism as a cause-and-effect model, a Cartesian machine with predictable and measurable functions in the physical world. While in some cases this model may hold true, physicians are baffled when the model fails. Despite Heisenberg's discovery that properties long thought to be both "predictable and measurable" are often neither, physicians have a persistent blind spot. In addition, though we have accomplished much, the science of medicine is still in its infancy and the great majority of the complex inner machinations of the human form have yet to be elucidated. Although many causes are still a mystery, we continue to rigidly apply a cause-and-effect model. In the modern medical world placebos should not work (they defy the cause-and-effect model), but they do. Physicians are mystified. Beta blockers administered during a heart attack should work (they fit the cause-and-effect model perfectly) but they don't, and again medical professionals are befuddled. The medical establishment plainly disbelieves; they shun placebos that work and use beta blockers that don't. The House of Medicine faithfully abides by models of thought that Heisenberg showed to be unreliable.

A common conflation of Heisenberg's principle with the impact of observation leads to the oft-noted principle that the act of observation unalterably impacts its object.* This, a related point, also has direct bearing on medicine: the stoic model of the modern physician that we endorse—the objective and uninvolved observer—does not exist. Our presence alters the path of illness and impacts the human experience. We are not detached

*The HUP dealt with the impossibility of simultaneous measurement of an atom's position and momentum. Measuring both simultaneously could lend certainty to a particle's behavior, but it cannot be done. The more precise the measurement of one, the less precise the measurement of the other. Many sources have confused this with the related fact that observation impacts the behavior of a particle being measured. In Heisenberg's case, the use of a photon to measure an atom's position changed the atom's momentum, therefore the act of observation impacted the answer. This is a related but separate point.

spectators nor should we be; we are an integral and powerful part of both illness and healing.

Gödel

A final, and globally more celebrated, revelation occurred just five years after Heisenberg's when twenty-five-year-old Kurt Gödel turned the world of mathematics and metamathematics on its ear with his paper "On Formally Undecidable Propositions of Principia Mathematica and Related Systems." The paper is as forbidding as it sounds, and is generally scrutinized only by the mathematical elite. However, much like the Heisenberg Uncertainty Principle and Bayes's Theorem, the essence of its conclusions is strikingly simple. Gödel demonstrated mathematically, and irrefutably, that logical consistency and truth are not synonymous.*

Gödel's proof had profound and far-reaching implications. Most significantly, Gödel's proof says that mathematics, the perfect language of science, retains its perfection only within the domain of mathematics. Pure logic allows one to arrive at an answer that is purely logical, but not necessarily an answer that is provably true. Gödel showed that a system that relies on purely logical deductions (an "axiomatic" system) may retain its

---

*The paper and its explanation are complex, but for our purposes here it is adequate to understand the following: by applying the rules of logic and deductive reasoning to sequences of statements, one can deduce a conclusion that is provably consistent—but not necessarily provably true. Mathematical systems that are entirely constructed based on logical deductions from a guiding set of accepted axioms (the field of geometry is such a system) were believed, after Whitehead and Russell's *Principia Mathematica* was published in 1910–1913, to be provably true. Gödel showed that while such systems may be consistent, it is not possible to verify their truth using any external measure. Thus they are "undecidable," as Gödel's title notes.

logic and consistency and may result in perfectly consistent conclusions. But despite their consistency within the system, those conclusions cannot be provably true because the only logic they follow is their own. Prior to Gödel it was believed that purely deductive reasoning from true statements could lead to statements that are also demonstrably and provably true. Gödel noted that there is no way to use external measures to demonstrate the truth of conclusions reached by such systems. When conclusions are not verifiably true, they are "undecidable."

For medicine and for science in general, it is a small step from here to the understanding that what works in theory may not work in practice, even when perfectly consistent scientific logic is employed. While deductive logic bears an esthetic that the scientific mind respects and seeks, the final product of this logic does not bear the infallibility, nor in many cases the applicability, that the esthetic implies. This lesson has played out in the House of Medicine's persistent but unsuccessful attempts to bring mathematical, logical precision to the treatment and diagnosis of human disease. The computers that print EKGs, for instance, mathematically interpret each tracing and offer a presumptive diagnosis. For years physicians and researchers believed that this could and would replace human judgment in the difficult field of EKG interpretation. But computers have failed to replace judgment, just as experts who have expounded on Gödel's proof predicted they would.[10] Despite human flaws, powerful computers could not (and still cannot) consistently match the diagnostic accuracy of a physician reading an EKG at the bedside. Similarly, neural networks devised to replace physician judgment for determining which patients are having heart attacks have failed. Light- and pattern-recognition systems developed to "assist" humans in reading X-rays for detecting cancer are no better than the human eye. Dozens of other attempts have all failed to supplant or even to consistently match the accuracy of human physicians in assessing human problems. Repeatedly, research in medicine has shown us that science and technology must be accompanied by human interpretation and human sensibility. Internal consistency, flawless in computer logic and mathematical systems, is not truth.

And yet what of medicine's inconsistencies? As I noted in chapter 5, physicians often disagree on the interpretation of EKGs, but it is not openly discussed with patients. It is perceived as failure, an awkward idiosyncrasy better left unsaid. But under the light of Bayes's Theorem, the Heisenberg Uncertainty Principle, and Gödel's proof, the flaw in these presumptions becomes apparent. Disagreement in the interpretation of EKGs does not indicate a failure of humans in interpreting science; it indicates a failure of science in interpreting humans. The problem is not in humans—it is in the machine.

What is the importance of these three revelations to human medicine? Science and the scientific technique have become a religion that modern man believes implicitly. The signs of this faith pervade our popular culture. Popular television shows currently tout science as the ultimate crime solver. Perhaps the Western world's best-known fictional detective, Sherlock Holmes, was renowned for his use of deductive technique. Infomercials use the words "scientifically proven" or "scientifically formulated" to sell products from creams to kitchen devices to get-rich-quick schemes. The word "science" is often used interchangeably with "truth" or "knowledge." The elevated status of science has become an integral part of the language of mass media, and an influential undercurrent in popular culture. Thus, science as religion, has come between patients and physicians.

Bayes's Theorem, Heisenberg's Principle, and Gödel's proof were all critiques of the scientific method's ability to arrive at truth, and together they offer a compelling deconstruction of the infallible vision of science that informs our patient-doctor bond. Bayes showed that the meaning and importance of the inquiry, the first step in the scientific method, were limited by context. Heisenberg showed that the veracity of the measurement, the next step in the scientific method, was often uncertain. And Gödel showed that no matter how central the inquiry or accurate the measurement, the truth of the conclusion, the final step in the scientific method, was not assured. Together these revelations demonstrate that the scientific method is highly imperfect, and the power of science is profoundly limited.

The shortcomings that these three discoveries predicted for medicine are not just a theory, or a point of dialectic. The impact of science on human life is increasingly limited. One study recently published in the *American Journal of Public Health* estimated that health-care progress during the 1990s, despite explosive growth in the use of CAT scans and MRIs, and a surge in the use of pills, may have extended or saved the lives of, at best, roughly one in every sixteen thousand people in the United States.* These findings stand in stark contrast to the results of a 1999 study that reported between 44,000 and 98,000 individuals die annually in this country due to medical errors—or about one in every four thousand people.[13] In our period of greatest

---

*The study[11] used a generous estimate. Non–health-care issues such as genetics, social circumstances, and behavior are presumed responsible for roughly 90 percent of mortality, however the authors of this study, in order to be as optimistic as possible about technological impacts, gave 100 percent of the credit of decreases in mortality rates to health-care technology advancement. If we presumed that only 10 percent of the credit goes to health-care advances then the number of lives saved per year would be close to the same number of people killed each year by a lightning strike or other natural disaster.[12]

health-care technology increases to date, four times more people died because of health-care errors than were saved because of advances.*

Why would these advances make such little difference? Partly because health care (as we practice it) is among the least important of the five domains that impact health and longevity. The other four, genetics, behavior, social circumstances (socioeconomic class), and environmental exposures, are estimated to be responsible for 90 percent of premature deaths. Behavioral issues alone, including alcohol misuse, smoking, poor diet, and physical inactivity, are responsible for the deaths of nearly a million people per year in the United States, or 40 percent of all those who die.[14]

This is not to say that modern medicine does not impact health. Antibiotics, vaccines, chemotherapy, and modern surgery have all played a critical role in increasing longevity and controlling disease, and I do not mean to minimize their importance. These advances save and extend lives every day. But these developments occurred more than fifty years ago and our society's reverence of them, as well as an increasing dependence on technological marvels like cell phones and computers, have altered the expectations of the modern mind. This cultural faith in science has crossed a threshold: our culture's faith that the scientific method will yield benefits has trumped the realization of those benefits. How? Consider the accepted standard for interpreting the results of placebo-controlled trials: when a drug or intervention is "equivalent to placebo" no one asks how good

---

*To do this calculation and to estimate the fraction (1 in 16,000) above, I used the 1996 census data reporting a population of 281 million in the United States. For the number of fatal medical errors I split the difference between the two estimated figures in the IOM report and used 71,000.

the placebo was. Even when the placebo was beneficial (as it often is), the intervention is considered a failure—despite being beneficial. When benefit is considered equivalent to no benefit, method has blatantly trumped outcome. Faith in the method to achieve benefit has become more important than achieving the benefit. Method has trumped outcome; theory has trumped reality.

Good or bad, wrong or right, this is the ethic of the scientific method. While it has a proper place in clinical trials, we as a culture have been unable to separate the laboratory from the clinic. We apply the standards and esthetics of scientific method to the practical world, where patients need benefits, not method. When scientific method is valued over outcome, as it routinely is now, theory is valued more than reality. Mammograms *should* find cancers early and save lives, so we endorse them. Antibiotics *should* help strep throat infections, so we prescribe them. Beta blockers *should* save lives during heart attacks, so we give them. These are sound theories. But hard evidence shows us that these theories have failed and that each is causing harm rather than good. Yet we continue to function as if each were robust, as if each theory had worked. Theory trumps reality.

For physicians this determined preference for science over sensibility is a tragic and costly weakness, and the flaw that leads to our secrecy. As faithful advocates of science, when there is conflict between theory and reality physicians have defended science, despite a promise to put patients first. Violating the Oath of Hippocrates, the oath that every physician has sworn, leads us to feel conflicted, alienated, and frustrated. These feelings are the heralds of secrecy. Our secrecy, a massive coping mechanism desperately erected and collectively maintained, is what we cling to. It is the outward expression of a broken promise.

•   •   •

Our breach is repairable. What has come between us? A religious belief in the perfection and power of science has come between us. Patients crave science instinctively and physicians defer to it reflexively. Modern culture has devalued the patient-doctor bond and medical truth, and encouraged the secrecy and separation needed to maintain this false religion. Physicians and patients are separated from within by a programmed, and shared, mentality. But we can question it and we can deprogram it. Change cannot be mandated, however, only chosen. We must choose to believe that humans are more important than science.

This change can be made without relinquishing the benefits of science and technology. Physicians and patients can continue to respect and believe in the power of science to save and improve lives, but we must also understand that it is the application of human principles and priorities to science that achieves true human benefit, and that immense benefits are available in nontechnological forms. An understanding of the array of benefits and their essential human context has evaded us, beginning from the early days of the Scientific Revolution, when the paths of physicians and patients began to diverge most sharply. Patients have remained passive, silent, and unquestioning while their physicians invoked and paraded "science." At the same time physicians have remained passive and silent as a culture of profit, consumerism, and mythical adulation of "science" has invaded and complicated the mission of real medicine. The reversal of this pattern will come when patients and physicians demand communication and truth from one another. When we do this, our secrecy will dissolve—there will be nothing to hide, and the Oath will be our guide. Truth will heal the breach.

The obstacles that remain, including our crumbling, un-Hippocratic health-care system, are surmountable. A paradigm shift will help to lift the weight of this broken system and refocus it on proactive care and appreciable benefits. When physicians and patients invest in human contact, believe in touch and word, and practice counsel and partnership, we will remove the vast burden of meaningless tests, unnecessary X-rays, and spurious pills. Egregious increases in spending on technologies that do not improve health will end, and real-world evidence of benefit will guide allocations. Expectations will be grounded, health will improve, needs will decrease, waits will be shorter, time will be longer, and we'll be healed by one another. We will be doctors and we will be patients.

With a revolutionary approach to his patients, Hippocrates became the father of medicine. His gift and his legacy are precisely what our modern medical system has spurned: the primacy of the patient above all else. As a culture we have misunderstood the role of science in medicine, and this false elevation has divided patients from doctors, allowing both to accept a bond that is not based on mutual trust. Hippocrates could not have envisioned the ways our practice has diverged from his own, both literally and figuratively. Patients and physicians have taken a step away from our history, away from our paragon, and ultimately away from one another. Hippocrates' belief in the bond, his respect for the mind/body, and his patient primacy are the foundations to which we must return, and from which a new paradigm can flourish. As always history is our guide: to reunite, we will have to embrace a paradigm that is both new, and very old.

A PATIENT GUIDE

On Knowing

Do not expect doctors to know everything. But do expect to understand what your doctor is saying. Physicians often lapse into jargon or speak in language that is difficult to understand. If you don't understand, ask questions. Push hard if necessary. Do not allow confusion to stand. When a physician continues to speak in ambiguities, it is often a sign that medical science doesn't have a concrete answer to your question. Ask if this is the case.

On What Works

Again, question everything. Many common and accepted interventions and practices don't work. Physicians sometimes recommend or prescribe measures that they know don't work, but more often they're unaware of the negative evidence behind accepted but fruitless health interventions. Take nothing for granted. If your physician doesn't have the answers, don't be afraid to ask them to find the answers.

On Agreement

Disagreement in medicine is frequently a sign of the limits of medical science. Schools of thought or differing interpretations often mean that there is no clear answer. A complete and honest conversation between a patient and doctor will clarify this. When doctors disagree, or when there appears to be room for discussion about the interpretation of a test, your first question should be whether this is a limitation of medical science or a matter of evidence. The question is a fair one, and you have the right to know which decisions are based on evidence and which are based on opinion.

On Communicating

Doctors are (remember this, please) humans. But they are humans who have been *trained to place the scientific pursuit of medicine above the connection between patient and doctor*. In rare instances, such as dire emergencies, this approach may have value, but for many if not most patients and conditions it leads to worse outcomes and poorer health than an approach that includes honest partnership. Nevertheless, the error pervades medical education and culture. Patients and doctors are taught to value the cold, unemotional, scientific model of medicine. It will take honesty, vulnerability, and openness on both ends of the stethoscope to break this barrier. Speak honestly and speak from the heart when you speak to your doctor, and you will have your best chance at receiving the same treatment.

On Tests

Medical tests should generally be ordered if and only if three conditions are present: a) a clear question can be articulated that the test can answer, b) there is a plan of action for the result, and c) a substantial chance exists that the answer may be either positive or negative. Examples:

1. Does your cough and fever represent pneumonia?
   - consider a chest X-ray to look for pneumonia
   - if the X-ray shows pneumonia, you'll start antibiotic therapy. If not, your infection is likely bronchitis, and antibiotics are more likely to harm than help.

2. Does your shortness of breath represent anemia (a low red-blood-cell count)?
   - consider checking a cell-blood count to look for anemia
   - if your counts are low, consider starting iron and undertaking a further workup for hidden sources of blood loss. If they're not low, the problem is not anemia.

3. Does your exertional chest pain represent possible coronary artery disease?
   - consider a stress test to look for indicators of coronary artery disease
   - if positive, you will likely need a cardiac catheterization to visualize your coronary arteries.

These are concrete questions with concrete plans, and each test clarifies the next step. Tests should not be ordered for no reason, or for vague reasons. Tests should not be ordered when your doctor already knows the answer with a reasonably high degree of certainty. Unnecessary testing, and reliance on testing, is how false-positives occur, how spending (on resources, time, and money) escalates, and how doctor and patient are separated.

On Unlearning

Most doctors are open to, and interested in, progress. It is an ominous sign when doctors are set in their ways and will not learn. Look for doctors who seem open to learning, and who are open to discussing the value of health interventions. Those willing to discuss are often willing to learn. The same goes, of course, for patients. You have learned as many or more falsehoods as your doctor has and you must be prepared to progress. It is correct, and indeed important, to have expectations and goals when you speak with your physician. You should be able to explicitly say why you are there and what you hope to gain from your visit. But be prepared to drop your expectations, be open to being wrong or being helped in ways that you weren't expecting. It is far more important to concentrate on what is right rather than on who is right.

Keep in mind that as evidence emerges in health care, practices change. Antibiotics should not be administered for the great majority of strep throats. This will be a surprise to most doctors, making it a challenging issue to raise and discuss. But doctors who are unwilling to discuss this with you are not likely to be interested in discussing the utility of many of the other interventions that you care about. If your doctor won't talk to you, or is unable to explain or research the rationale behind common interventions that you inquire about, it may be time to switch doctors.

On Placebos and Meaning

The most important revelation that arises from our understanding of placebos and meaning is that the mind and the body are not separate entities. Treating patients as partners in care, as humans with a social, physical, and emotional milieu, maximizes health and health care. Communication and a sense of being cared for are important components of the healing and health processes. Health-care interventions will work better when the doctor and patient are working in tandem, and pills and procedures will become less important (and occasionally unnecessary). Find a doctor who understands that the human connection is a health-care tool, and one that is often more powerful and more important than any pill.

On the NNT

The Number Needed to Treat is a tool that translates. It is understandable across levels of education and across cultures and subcultures. Most physicians don't use the NNT, but they should, or else they should have a tool just like it. This is a relatively new way of communicating and there's nothing wrong with a physician who hasn't communicated in this way before. But there is something wrong with a physician who refuses to learn about these ways of communicating now. Embedded in the NNT is an honest assessment of the value of health-care interventions. Ask for it. In fact, demand it. You need to know how much the health interventions you undertake have the potential to help you, and which ones matter most. This is basic literacy for patients and doctors. In the long run both you and your doctor will be happy you did.

On a New Paradigm

A new way of thinking about medicine is up to all of us, and given the current trajectory of modern medicine, a new paradigm is both imperative and inevitable. But it can't be mandated or legislated. It's a choice. If you choose to believe in health care that is honest about its strengths and weaknesses, and clear about its certainties and uncertainties, then your doctor will, too.

ACKNOWLEDGMENTS

At the risk of trite cliché, first and foremost I thank my mother. She is my brilliant editor and my tireless cheerleader, and she is the reason that this book exists. She is good and she is right.

Binky Urban saw a sculpture inside this block of marble. Binky is the talent among the talent, and her vision is the gift that marks her. I will forever be profoundly grateful to have been an unlikely beneficiary. Thank you, Binky.

Nan Graham, Nan Graham, Nan Graham. Nan and Susan Moldow also have the gift and graciously accepted this stone. Thank you to Jim Morgan, whose patience is impressive and whose skill as an editor and writer are apparent here. To Samantha Martin: I will not be able to properly convey my gratitude. Samantha is brilliant, perceptive, and probing, and these pages (all of them) reflect her work. Meetings and diet cola in the library with Samantha were where my writer's eyesight began to find focus. And in case I didn't say it before: Nan Graham, Nan Graham, Nan Graham.

My sister, Andrea Newman, is a deeply gifted writer. Anything that I have, anything that I am, anything that I have done, is a reflection of her and her talent and her help. This book is no different. My father believes in me, and his generosity of spirit and dedication to advocacy are not just guiding principles within this book, they are a reason for it.

Leslie Marnett has been my strength and my secret editor. She is Beauty, and she is the reality and the gift that keeps these pages grounded and true. Beauty's time, love, and strength are all here, and she reminds me every day to walk rather than simply to talk. Love is a many-splendored thing. For truth, Beauty.

Lucas Miller, a brilliant writer and lifelong friend to whom I owe more than I know how to say, sculpted this book and gave me the gift of his concentration, criticism, and conversation. Reading the cave drawings of friends (and others) is the burden that all serious writers are, quite unfairly, asked to bear. Luke gracefully accepted this burden. This is unsurprising, for Luke and Jen are two of the most socially graceful humans I have ever known. They and Dick and Joan are all an inspiration for this book.

Many doctors have played a role, too many to list. Abby Wolfson, my friend, my travel companion, and my EM mentor, was yet another secret editor. Abby, more than anyone, suffered my resistance with tolerance and time, as he always has. And as it always has, it improved me. It also improved the book. Cliff Callaway, a genius-level researcher and a profoundly good human, is as dedicated to the truth as anyone I have ever met. I am lucky to have worked with him. I would like to believe that his passionate search for truth is emulated in this book. Other excellent doctors who have, knowingly and unknowingly, played an important role in this book include Dan Wiener, Ian Green-wald, Vince Verdile, and Henry Pohl. And of course, the enduring goodness of the men and women, doctors and all, of the 344th.

NOTES

CHAPTER 1: WE DON'T KNOW

1. Moayyedi, P. 2006. Can the clinical history distinguish between organic and functional dyspepsia? *JAMA* 295 (13): 1566–76.
2. Sánchez-Guerrero, J., G. A. Colditz, E. W. Karlson, et al. 1995. Silicone breast implants and the risk of connective-tissue diseases and symptoms. *NEJM* 332 (25): 1666–70; Silverman, B. G., S. L. Brown, R. A. Bright, et al. 1996. Reported complications of silicone gel breast implants: An epidemiologic review. *Ann Intern Med* 124 (8): 744–56; Janowsky, E. C., L. L. Kupper, B. S. Hulka. 2000. Meta-analyses of the relation between silicone breast implants and the risk of connective-tissue diseases *NEJM* 342 (11): 781–90.
3. Hammond, S. R., J. G. McLeod, K. S. Millingen, et al. 1988. The epidemiology of multiple sclerosis in three Australian cities: Perth, Newcastle and Hobart. *Brain* 111: 1–25; Kuroiwa, Y., H. Shibasaki, M. Ikeda. 1983. Prevalence of multiple sclerosis and its north–south gradient in Japan. *Neuroepidemiology* 2: 62–69; Kurtzke, J. F., G. W. Beebe, J. E. Norman. 1979. Epidemiology of multiple sclerosis in U.S. veterans. I. Race, sex and geographic distribution. *Neurology* 29: 1228–35; Skegg, D. C., P. A. Corwin, R. S. Craven, J. A. Malloch, M. Pollock. 1987. Occurrence of multiple sclerosis in the north and south of New Zealand. *J Neurol Neurosurg Psychiatry* 50: 134–39.
4. Jarvik, J. G., R. A. Deyo. 2002. Diagnostic Evaluation of low back pain with emphasis on imaging. *Annals of Internal Medicine* 137 (7): 586–97.
5. Porchet, F., et al. 1999. The assessment of appropriate indications for laminectomy. *Journal of Bone & Joint Surgery* (British volume) 81 (2): 234–39.

6. Weber, H. 1983. Lumbar disc herniation: A controlled, prospective study with ten years of observation. *Spine* 8: 131–40; Loupasis, G. A., et al. 1999. Seven-to-20-year outcome of lumbar discectomy. *Spine* 24 (22): 2313–17.

7. Weinstein, J. N. 2006. Surgical vs. nonoperative treatment for lumbar disk herniation. The Spine Patient Outcomes Research Trial (SPORT): A randomized trial. *JAMA* 296 (20): 2441–50.

8. Jones, W. H. S. 1931. *Hippocrates (Volume IV)* (Cambridge, MA: Harvard University Press), xxiii.

CHAPTER 2: IT DOESN'T WORK

1. Lubitz, J. B. 1993. Trends in Medicare payments in the last year of life. *New England Journal of Medicine* 328 (15): 1092–96.

2. Nichol, G. 1996. Effectiveness of emergency medical services for victims of out-of-hospital cardiac arrest: A meta-analysis. *Annals of Emergency Medicine* 27 (6): 700–710. (From multiple large EMS systems, 93 percent failure.)

3. Stiell, I. 2004. Advanced cardiac life support in out-of-hospital cardiac arrest. *NEJM* 351: 647–56. (From Ottawa, Canada, a study of more than ten thousand cardiac arrests, 95 percent failure.)

4. Lombardi, G., et al. 1994. Outcome of out-of-hospital cardiac arrest in New York City. The Pre-Hospital Arrest Survival Evaluation (PHASE) Study. *JAMA* 271 (9): 678–83. (More recently presented, currently unpublished data from New York City appear to show a rising success rate in the past ten years, from 1 percent to about 2 percent.)

5. Valenzuela, T. D., et al. 2000. Outcomes of rapid defibrillation by security officers after cardiac arrest in casinos. *NEJM* 343 (17): 1206–09.

6. Stiell, I. 2004. Advanced cardiac life support in out-of-hospital cardiac arrest. *NEJM* 351: 647–56.

7. Poses, R. M., et al. 1985. The accuracy of experienced physicians' probability estimates for patients with sore throats: Implications for decision making. *JAMA* 254: 925–29.

8. Hirschmann, J. V. 2002. Antibiotics for common respiratory tract infections in adults. *Arch Int Med* 162 (3): 256–64.

9. National Hospital Ambulatory Care Survey statistics (NHAMCS), 2002. Outpatient Department Summary. *Advance Data From Vital and Health Statistics,* 2004. 340; 1–36. 345; 1–36. 346; 1–44.

10. Straus, S. E., et al. 2002. *Evidence-Based Acute Medicine* (London: Churchill Livingstone).

11. Peterson, M. "What's Black and White and Sells Medicine?" *New York Times*, August 27, 2000.

12. *Prescription Drug Therapies: Reducing Costs and Improving Outcomes.* Research in Action, Issue 8. AHRQ Publication No. 02–0045. September 2002. AHRQ, Rockville, MD. http://www.ahrq.gov/qual/rxtherapies/rxria.htm.

13. AHRQ document *Management of Acute Otitis Media.* Summary, Evidence Report/Technology Assessment: Number 15, June 2000, http://www.ahrq.gov/clinic/epcsums/otitisum.htm.

14. Schroeder, et al. 2002. Systematic review of randomized controlled trials of over-the-counter cough medicine for acute cough in adults. *BMJ* 324 (7333): 329–34; Schroeder, et al. 2002. Should we advise parents to administer over-the-counter cough medicines for acute cough? Systematic review of randomized controlled trials. *Archives of Disease in Childhood* 86 (3): 170–75.

15. Eccles, R. 1996. Codeine, cough, and upper respiratory infection. *Pulmonary Pharmacology* 9 (5–6): 293–97; Bolser, D. C. 2006. Cough suppressant and pharmacologic protussive therapy. ACCP evidence-based clinical practice guidelines. *Chest* 128: 239S–248S.

16. See http://www.robitussin.ca. Accessed 5/07.

17. See http://www.robitussin.com/cough/cough_la.asp. Accessed 5/07.

18. Hall, F. M. 2007. Breast imaging and computer-aided detection. *NEJM* 356 (14): 1464–66.

19. "Spotting Breast Cancer: Doctors Are Weak Link," *New York Times*, June 22, 2002.

20. Fletcher, S. W., et al. 2003. Mammographic screening for breast cancer. *NEJM* 348 (17): 1672–80.

21. Elmore, J. G., et al. 1998. Ten-year risk of false positive screening mammograms and clinical breast examinations. *NEJM* 338 (16): 1089–96.

22. Lerman, C. 1991. Psychological and behavioral implications of abnormal mammograms. *Ann Int Med* 114 (8): 657–61.

23. Feig, S. A. 1996. Assessment of radiation risk from screening mammography. *Cancer* 77: 818–22.

24. Fletcher, S. W., et al. 2003. Mammographic screening for breast cancer. *NEJM* 348 (17): 1672–80.

25. Shaneyfelt, T. M., M. F. Mayo-Smith, J. Rothwangl. 1999. Are guidelines following guidelines? The methodological quality of clinical practice guidelines in the peer-reviewed medical literature. *JAMA* 281 (20): 1900–05.

26. Schilling, F. H. 2002. Neuroblastoma screening at one year of age. *NEJM* 346 (14): 1047–53; Woods, W. G. 2002. Screening of infants and mortality due to neuroblastoma. *NEJM* 346 (14): 1041–46.

27. Epstein, S. S. 2001. Dangers and unreliability of mammography: Breast examination is a safe, effective, and practical alternative. *International Journal of Health Services* 31 (3): 606–15.
28. Sanchez-Menegay, et al. 1992. Patient expectations and satisfaction with medical care for upper respiratory infections. *Journal of General Internal Medicine* 7 (4): 432–34; Hamm, et al. 1996. Antibiotics and respiratory infections: Are patients more satisfied when expectations are met? *Journal of Family Practice* 43 (1): 56–62; Ong, S., et al. 2007. Antibiotic use for emergency department patients with upper respiratory infections: Prescribing practices, patient expectations, and patient satisfaction. *Annals of Emergency Medicine* 50 (3): 213–20.
29. See http://www.fda.gov/cder/ddmac/globalsummit2003. 8/6/07.
30. Harris, R., K. N. Lohr. 2002. Screening for prostate cancer: An update of the evidence for the U.S. Preventive Services Task Force. *Ann Intern Med* 137: 917–29.
31. The International Early Lung Cancer Action Program Investigators. 2006. Survival of patients with stage I lung cancer detected on CT screening. *NEJM* 355: 1763–71.
32. Bach, et al. 2007. Computed tomography screening and lung cancer outcomes. *JAMA* 297 (9): 953–61.

CHAPTER 3: WE DON'T AGREE

1. Gadsboll, N. 1989. Symptoms and signs of heart failure in patients with myocardial infarction: Reproducibility and relationship to chest X-ray, radionuclide ventriculography and right heart catheterization. *European Heart Journal* 10 (11): 1017–28.
2. Hickan, D. H. 1985. Systematic bias in recording the history in patients with chest pain. *J Chronic Dis* 38: 91–100.
3. Davies, L. G. 1958. Observer variation in reports of electrocardiograms. *Br Heart J* 20: 153–61.
4. Willems, J. L. 1991. The diagnostic performance of computer programs for the interpretation of electrocardiograms. *NEJM* 325: 1767–73.
5. Spiteri, M. A., et al. 1988. Reliability in eliciting physical signs in examination of the chest. *Lancet* 1: 873–75 (note on interpretation: Kappa values ranged from 0.1 to 0.51 ["poor" and "fair"], and raw agreement ranged from 63 to 85 percent in this study of multiple lung conditions, including pneumonia); Wipf, J. E. 1999. Diagnosing pneumonia by physical examination: Relevant or relic? *Arch Int Med* 159 (10): 1082–87. (Note on interpretation: The Kappa value averaged 0.51. The best val-

ues were seen for "rales," a crackling sound in the lung. Half of the six calculated Kappa values for rales were "moderate" or worse, half were in the lowest range of "good." All other sounds were poor, fair, or moderate.)

6. Robinson, P. J. A. 1999. Variation between experienced observers in the interpretation of accident and emergency radiographs. *Br J Rad* 72 (856): 323–30.

7. Garland, L. H. 1949. On the scientific evaluation of diagnostic procedures. *Radiology* 52: 309–28.

8. Pryse-Phillips, W. E., et al. 1997. Guidelines for the diagnosis and management of migraine in clinical practice. Canadian Headache Society. *Can Med Assoc J* 156: 1273–87.

9. Kelly, A. M. 2000. Migraine: Pharmacotherapy in the emergency department. *J Accid Emerg Med* 17: 241–45.

10. Lexchin, J., et al. 2003. Pharmaceutical industry sponsorship and research outcome and quality: Systematic review. *BMJ* 326: 1167–70.

11. Lipton, R. B., et al. 2004. Double-blind clinical trials of oral triptans vs other classes of acute migraine medication—a review. *Cephalalgia* 24 (5): 321–32.

12. Friedman, B. W., et al. 2005. A trial of metoclopramide versus sumatriptan for the emergency department treatment of migraines. *Neurology* 64 (3): 463–68.

CHAPTER 4: WE DON'T TALK

1. Safran, D. G. 2003. Defining the future of primary care: What can we learn from patients? *Ann Int Med* 138 (3): 248–55.

2. Rosenthal, et al. 2005. White coat, mood indigo—Depression in medical school. *NEJM* 353 (11): 1085–88.

3. Ramirez, A. J., et al. 1995. Burnout and psychiatric disorder among cancer clinicians. *British Journal of Cancer* 71 (6): 1263–69.

4. Mayer, R. J., et al. 1998. Report on the task force of end of life issues. Presidential Symposium, 34th Annual Meeting of the ASCO, Los Angeles, May 1998.

5. Bachman, L. M., et al. 2003. Accuracy of Ottawa ankle rules to exclude fractures of the ankle and midfoot: Systematic review. *BMJ* 326 (7386): 417–23.

6. Graham, I. D., et al. 2001. Awareness and use of the Ottawa ankle and knee rules in 5 countries: Can publication alone be enough to change practice? *Ann Emerg Med* 37 (3): 259–66.

7. Wilson, D. E., et al. 2002. Evaluation of patient satisfaction and outcomes after assessment for acute ankle injuries. *Am J Emerg Med* 20 (1): 18–22.

8. Gallagher, T. H., et al. 1997. How do physicians respond to patients' requests for costly, unindicated services? *J Gen Int Med* 12 (11): 663–68.

9. Cooke, M., D. M. Irby, W. Sullivan, et al. 2006. American medical education 100 years after the Flexner Report. *NEJM* 355 (13): 1339–44.

10. Gawande, A. 2005. Naked. *NEJM* 353 (7): 645–48.

11. Betancourt, J. R. 2004. Becoming a physician: cultural competence—marginal or mainstream movement? *NEJM* 351 (10): 953–55.

12. Fox, R. C. 2005. Cultural competence and the culture of medicine. *NEJM* 353 (13): 1316–19.

13. Zuger, A. 2004. Dissatisfaction with Medical Practice. *NEJM* 350 (1): 69–75; Safran, D. G. 2003. Defining the future of primary care: What can we learn from patients? *Ann Int Med* 138 (3): 248–55.

14. Levinson, W., et al. 1997. Physician-patient communication: The relationship with malpractice claims among primary care physicians and surgeons *JAMA* 277 (7): 553–55; Hickson, G. B., et al. 1992. Factors that prompted families to file medical malpractice claims following perinatal injuries. *JAMA* 267 (10): 1359–63; Kraman, S. S. 1999. Risk management: Extreme honesty may be the best policy. *Ann Int Med* 131 (12): 963–67.

CHAPTER 5: WE PREFER TESTS

1. Zuger, A. 2004. Dissatisfaction with medical practice. *N Engl J Med* 350: 69–75.

2. Haas, J. S., et al. 2000. Is the professional satisfaction of general internists associated with patient satisfaction? *J Gen Intern Med* 15: 122–28.

3. Mechanic, D., et al. 2001. Are patients' office visits with physicians getting shorter? *N Engl J Med* 344: 198–204.

4. American Heart Association. Heart disease and stroke statistics—2004 update. Dallas (TX): American Heart Association, 2003.

5. Ashley, E. A., J. Myers, V. Froelicher. 2000. Exercise testing in clinical medicine. *Lancet* 356 (9241): 1592–97.

6. Bastian, L. A., K. Nanda, V. Hasselblad, D. L. Simel. 1998. Diagnostic efficiency of home pregnancy test kits: A meta-analysis. *Archives of Family Medicine* 7 (5): 465–69.

7. Elmore, J. G., et al. 1998. Ten-year risk of false positive screening mammograms and clinical breast exams. *N Engl J Med* 338 (16): 1089–96; Elmore, J. G., et al. 2005. Screening for breast cancer. *JAMA* 293 (10): 1245–56.

8. Rheumatic fever and rheumatic heart disease. Report of a WHO Study

Group. World Health Organization, Geneva, 1988 (Technical Report Series No. 764).

9. Jauhar, S. 2006. Becoming a physician: The demise of the physical exam. *N Engl J Med* 354: 548–51.

CHAPTER 6: WE WON'T UNLEARN
(THE PSEUDOAXIOMS)

1. Straus, S. E., et al. 2002. *Evidence-Based Acute Medicine* (London: Churchill Livingstone).
2. Denny, F. W., et al. 1950. Prevention of rheumatic fever. Treatment of the preceding streptococcic infection. *JAMA* 143 (2): 151–53; Brink, W. R., et al. 1951. Effect of penicillin and aureomycin on the natural course of streptococcal tonsillitis and pharyngitis. *Am J Med* 10: 300–308; Wannamaker, L. W., et al. 1951. Prophylaxis of acute rheumatic fever by treatment of the preceding streptococcal infection with various amounts of depot penicillin. *Am J Med* 10: 673–94; Denny, F. W., et al. 1953. Comparative effects of penicillin, aureomycin, and terramycin on streptococcal tonsillitis and pharyngitis. *Pediatrics* 11: 7–14; Chamovitz, R., et al. 1954. Prevention of rheumatic fever by treatment of previous streptococcal infection. *New Engl J of Med* 251: 466–71; Catanzaro F., A. Morris, R. Chamovitz, et al. 1954. Symposium on rheumatic fever and rheumatic heart disease. The role of streptococcus in the pathogenesis of rheumatic fever. *Am J Med* 17: 749–56.
3. Webb, K. 2000. Use of a high-sensitivity rapid strep test without culture confirmation of negative results: 2 years' experience. *Journal of Family Practice* 49 (1): 34–38.
4. MMWR, Summary of Notifiable Diseases, 1997; 46 (54): 1–87.
5. Bronze, M. S. 1996. The reemergence of serious group A strep infections and acute rheumatic fever. *Am J Med Sci* 311 (1): 41–54.
6. Zoltie, N., M. P. Cust. 1986. Analgesia in the acute abdomen. *Annals of the Royal College of Surgeons, England* 68: 209–10; Sumant, R. R., et al. 2006. Do opiates affect the clinical evaluation of patients with acute abdominal pain? *JAMA* 296: 1764–74.
7. Bunnell, S., *Surgery of the Hand*, 3rd ed., vol. 1 (Philadelphia: J. B. Lippincott, 1956).
8. Waterbrook, et al. 2007. Is epinephrine harmful when used with anesthetics for digital nerve blocks? *Ann Emerg Med* 50 (4): 472–75.
9. Chapter XV in *Sex, Society and the Individual,* edited by A. P. Phillay and Albert Ellis, published by *International Journal of Sexology,* Bombay, India, 1953, 118–20.

10. Tiedemann, F. *Tabulae nervorum uteri* (Heidelberg, 1822); Krantz, K. 1959. Innervation of the human vulva and vagina. *Obstet Gynecol* 12: 382–96; Hilliges, M., et al. 1995. Innervation of the human vaginal mucosa as revealed by PGP 9.5 immunohistochemistry. *Acta Anat* 153 (2): 119–26.

11. Addiego, F., et al. 1981. Female ejaculation: A case study. *J Sex Res* 17: 1–13; Goldberg, D. C., et al. 1983. The Grafenberg spot and female ejaculation: A review of initial hypotheses. *Journal of Sex & Marital Therapy* 9 (1): 27–37.

12. Zaviacic, M. 2002. The G-spot. *Am J of Obst & Gyn* 187 (2): 519–20.

13. Pickering, G. W. 1956. The purpose of medical education. *BMJ* 2: 113–16.

14. Poynard, T., et al. 2002. Truth survival in clinical research: An evidence-based requiem? *Ann Intern Med* 136: 888–95.

CHAPTER 7: WE'RE MISSING THE MEANING
(THE PLACEBO PARADOX)

1. Moseley, J. B. 2002. A controlled trial of arthroscopic surgery for osteoarthritis of the knee. *New Engl J Med* 347 (2): 81–88.

2. Talbot, M. The placebo prescription. *New York Times Magazine,* January 9, 2000.

3. Dimond, E. G. 1960. Comparison of internal mammary ligation and sham operation for angina pectoris. *Am J Card* 5: 483–86; Cobb, L. 1959. An evaluation of internal mammary artery ligation by a double blind technic. *New Engl J Med* 260 (22): 1115–18.

4. Freed, C. R., et al. 2001. Transplantation of embryonic dopamine neurons for severe Parkinson's disease. *NEJM* 344 (10): 710–19.

5. De la Fuente-Fernandez, R., et al. 2001. Expectation and dopamine release: Mechanism of the placebo effect in Parkinson's disease. *Science.* 293: 1164–66.

6. Moerman, D. E. 2002. *Meaning, Medicine, and the "Placebo Effect"* (Cambridge, U.K.: Cambridge University Press); Kaptchuk, T. 2002. The placebo effect in alternative medicine: Can the performance of a healing ritual have clinical significance? *Ann Int Med* 136 (11): 817–25.

7. Cabot, R. 1903. The use of truth and falsehood in medicine: An experimental study. *Am Med* 5: 344–49.

8. Kaptchuk, T. J. 1998. Powerful placebo: The dark side of the randomized controlled trial. *Lancet* 351 (9117): 1722–25.

9. Beecher, H. K. 1961. Surgery as placebo. A quantitative study of bias. *JAMA* 176: 1102–7.

10. Moerman, D. E. 2002. Deconstructing the placebo effect and finding the meaning response. *Ann Int Med* 136 (6): 471–76.
11. Kaptchuk, T. 2002. The placebo effect in alternative medicine: Can the performance of a healing ritual have clinical significance? *Ann Int Med* 136 (11): 917–25.
12. Linde, K. 2005. Acupuncture for patients with migraine. A randomized controlled trial. *JAMA* 293 (17): 2118–25.
13. Bienenfeld, L. 1996. The placebo effect in cardiovascular disease. *Am Heart J* 132 (6): 1207–21; Walsh, B. T. 2002. Placebo response in studies of major depression. *JAMA* 287 (14): 1840–47.

CHAPTER 8: YOU'RE A NUMBER (THE "NNT")

1. Antithrombotic Trialists' Collaboration. 2002. Collaborative meta-analysis of randomized trials of anti-platelet therapy for prevention of death, myocardial infarction, and stroke in high risk patients. *BMJ* 324 (7329): 71–86.
2. Elwood, P. 2005. For and against. Aspirin for everyone older than 50? *BMJ* 330: 1440–41.
3. WebMD referral: http://rxlist.com/top200.htm.
4. Mulrow, C. 2005. Pharmacotherapy for hypertension in the elderly. *Cochrane Database of Systematic Reviews* 3.
5. 2005 American Heart Association Guidelines for Cardiopulmonary Resuscitation and Emergency Cardiovascular Care. Part 8: Stabilization of the Patient with Acute Coronary Syndromes. *Circulation* (2005): 112:IV89–IV110.
6. Hjalmarson, A. 1983. The Goteborg metoprolol trial: Effects on mortality and morbidity in acute myocardial infarction: Limitation of infarct size by beta blockers and its potential role for prognosis. *Circulation* 67 (suppl I): I26–I32; the MIAMI Trial Research Group. 1985. Metoprolol in acute myocardial infarction (MIAMI). A randomised placebo-controlled international trial. *European Heart Journal* 6: 199–226; Randomised trial of intravenous atenolol among 16,027 cases of suspected acute myocardial infarction: ISIS-1. First International Study of Infarct Survival Collaborative Group. *Lancet* (1986) 2: 57–66.
7. Pollack, C. V. 2006. Application of the TIMI risk score for unstable angina and non-ST elevation acute coronary syndrome to an unselected emergency department chest pain population academic emergency medicine 13 (1): 13–18.

8. Juni, P., et al. 2002. Are selective COX 2 inhibitors superior to traditional nonsteroidal anti-inflammatory drugs? Adequate analysis of the CLASS trial indicates that this may not be the case. *BMJ* 324: 1287–88.

9. Curfman, G. D., et al. 2000. Expression of concern: "Comparison of upper gastrointestinal toxicity of rofecoxib and naproxen in patients with rheumatoid arthritis" [*N Engl J Med* 343: 1520–28. *N Engl J Med* 353 (26): 2813–14].

10. Prosser, H., et al. 2003. General practitioner's decisions to prescribe new drugs. The importance of who says what. *Family Practice* 20 (1): 61.

11. Wazana, A. 2000. Physicians and the pharmaceutical industry: Is a gift ever just a gift? *JAMA* 283: 373–80.

12. See http://www.fda.gov/cder/ddmac/globalsummit2003/.

13. Baciu, A., et al. 2006. *The Future of Drug Safety: Promoting and Protecting the Health of the Public* (Washington, D.C.: National Academies Press).

14. Smith, S. W. 2007. Sidelining safety—the FDA's inadequate response to the IOM. *NEJM* 357 (10): 960–63.

15. Writing Group for the WHI Investigators. 2002. Risks and benefits of estrogen plus progestin in healthy postmenopausal women: Principal results from the Women's Health Initiative randomized controlled trial. *JAMA* 288 (3): 321–33.

16. MacLennan, A. H. 2007. Oral oestrogen and combined oestrogen/ progestogen therapy versus placebo for hot flushes. Cochrane Menstrual Disorders and Subfertility Group. *Cochrane Database of Systematic Reviews 3*.

17. Hashish, I., et al. 1988. Reduction of postoperative pain and swelling by ultrasound treatment: A placebo effect. *Pain* 33: 303–11.

18. Randomized trial of intravenous streptokinase, oral aspirin, both, or neither among 17,187 cases of suspected acute myocardial infarction: ISIS-2. ISIS-2 (Second International Study of Infarct Survival) Collaborative Group. *Journal of the American College of Cardiology* (1988) 12 (6 Suppl A): 3A–13A.

CHAPTER 8: TABLE CREDITS

1. Harris, R. 2002. Screening for prostate cancer: An update of the evidence for US preventive services task force. *Annals of Internal Medicine* 137: 917–29.

2. Jolliffe, J. A. 2000. Cochrane. Exercise-based rehabilitation for coronary artery disease. *Cochrane Database of Systematic Reviews 4*.

3. Hooper, L. 2003. Advice to reduce dietary salt for prevention of cardiovascular disease. *Cochrane Database of Systematic Reviews 1*.

4. Critchley, J. 2003. Smoking cessation for the secondary prevention of coronary heart disease. *Cochrane Database of Systematic Reviews 4*.

5. Roberts, L. 1997. Intercessory prayer for alleviation of ill health. *Cochrane Database of Systematic Reviews* 4.

CHAPTER 9: A NEW OLD PARADIGM

1. Catlin, A., C. Cowan, M. Hartman, S. Heffler. 2008. National health spending in 2006: A year of change for prescription drugs. *Health Aff* 27: 14–29.
2. Anderson, G. F., B. K. Frogner, U. E. Reinhardt. 2007. Health spending in OECD countries in 2004: An update. *Health Aff* 26 (5): 1481–89.
3. Schroeder, S. 2007. We can do better—improving the health of the American people. *NEJM* 357 (12): 1221–28.
4. Gawande, A. "The Checklist," *The New Yorker,* December 10, 2007.
5. Ward, E., et al. 2007. Association of Insurance with Cancer Care Utilization and Outcomes. *CA: A Cancer Journal for Clinicians,* DOI: 10.3322/CA.2007.0011.
6. Kennedy, B. P., et al. 1996. Income distribution and mortality: Cross sectional ecological study of the Robin Hood index in the United States. *BMJ* 312: 1004–7; Lynch, J. W., et al. 1998. Income inequality and mortality in metropolitan areas of the United States. *Am J Public Health* 88: 1074–80.
7. Hsia, R. Y., et al. Decreasing reimbursements for outpatient emergency department visits across payer groups from 1996 to 2004. *Ann Emerg Med,* DOI: 10.1016/j.annemergmed.2007.08.009.
8. Kellerman, A. 2006. Crisis in the emergency department. *N Engl J Med* 355 (13): 1300–3.
9. Schoen, C., et al. 2004. Primary care and health system performance: adults' experiences in five countries. *Health Affairs* (Millwood), http://content .healthaffairs.org/cgi/content/full/hlthaff.w4.487/DC1.
10. Nagel, E., J. R. Newman. 2001 (1958). *Gödel's Proof* (New York: New York University Press).
11. Woolfe, S., et al. 2004. The health impact of resolving racial disparities: An analysis of US mortality data. *Am J Pub Health* 94 (12): 2078–81.
12. National Safety Council. 2007. What are the odds of dying? http://www .nsc.org/lrs/statinfo/odds.htm.
13. Kohn, L. T., Corrigan, M. S. Donaldson. 1999. *To Err Is Human: Building a Safer Health System* (Washington, D.C.: National Academy Press).
14. Mokdad, A. H., et al. 2004. Actual causes of death in the U.S., 2000. *JAMA* 291: 1238–45.

INDEX

ABOUT THE AUTHOR

A native New Yorker, David Newman studied philosophy at SUNY Binghamton and received his medical degree from Albany Medical College. At thirty-five, as a major in the army reserve, he was deployed to Iraq in 2005 where he received an Army Commendation Medal for his work with the 344th Combat Support Hospital. Published regularly in biomedical journals, Newman currently runs a clinical research program and teaches at Columbia University and in the Department of Emergency Medicine at St. Luke's–Roosevelt Hospital Center in New York City.

Breinigsville, PA USA
07 April 2011
259326BV00005B/3/P